TALI SHINE
STEPH ADAMS

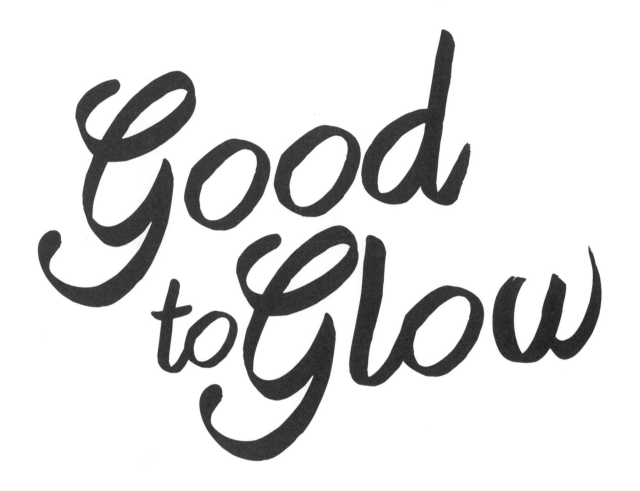

Good to Glow

FEEL GOOD FOOD

teNeues

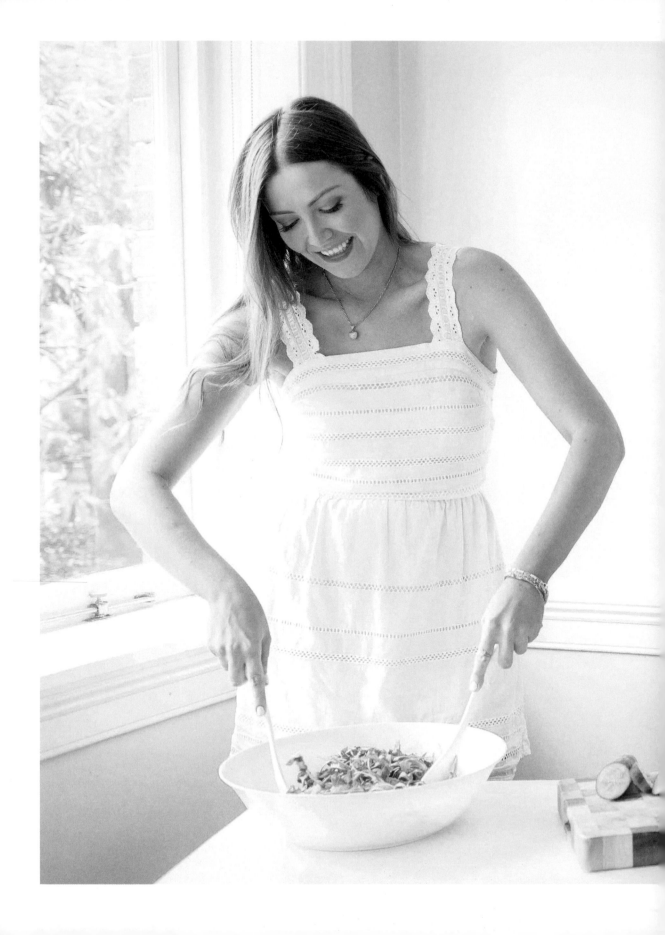

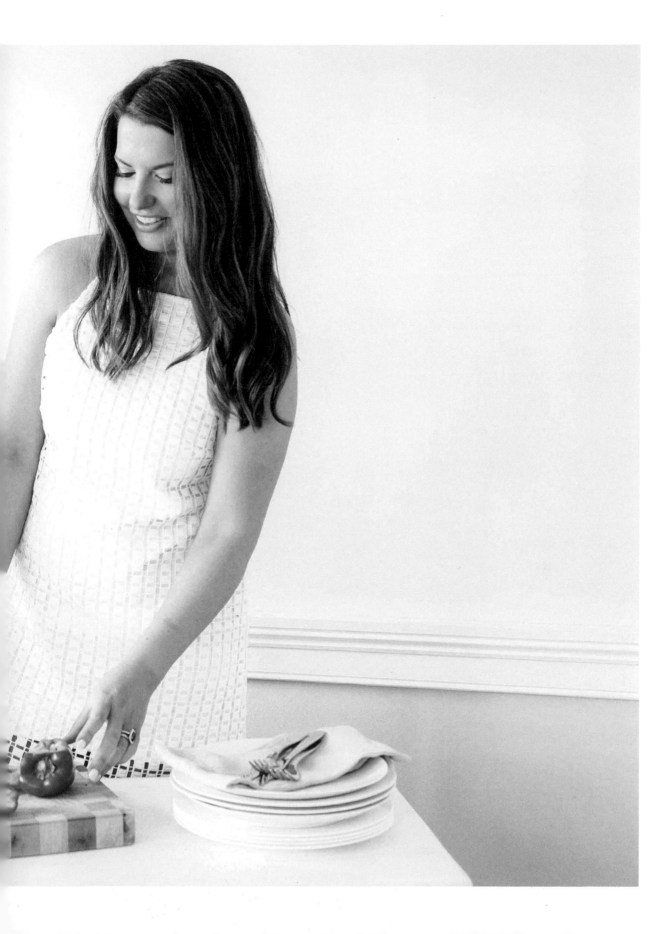

TABLE OF CONTENTS

WELCOME TO GOOD TO GLOW

I have been an advocate for clean eating, green juices, and healthy living for as long as I can remember. I never had to watch my weight or worry about pimples or low energy. Then one day suddenly everything changed. My body shifted out of whack. I had extra niggling pounds that I could not get rid of no matter how many gym classes I took. I had outbreaks on my previously clear skin, waning energy, and a permanently foggy head.

I went from doctor, to specialist, to nutritionist, to dermatologist without any solution or improvement. My friends would say, "You really should weigh less than you do considering your portions and the amount of time you spend at the gym."

It was only when I really cleaned up my diet—initially cutting out even the small amount of treats I allowed myself—and committed to Alkaline living that the symptoms changed. I started feeling more energetic, I did not have constant head-fog and didn't need a nap in the middle of the day. My skin cleared and I was able to get back to my previous weight!

The idea behind *Good to Glow* came about as a way to share inspiring, easy, and delicious recipes to cook at home, as well as information about amazing cafes in every corner of the globe so you, too, can look and feel your healthy best.

I hope you enjoy!

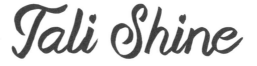

There is no such thing as perfection. This book is not about being perfect, but about eating a balanced diet so you can lead a healthy life and look your glowing best!

After modeling for more than eight years, I had tried every diet known to man. I know firsthand that diets do not work. The moment you deprive yourself of something is the moment you will want it more. The best answer to a long life of good health is to lose the diet mindset and establish a well-balanced eating plan, incorporate exercise into your daily routine, and make these changes slowly.

It has taken me years to realize the importance of good nutrition and why we need to keep our body free of toxins. In 2009, I moved to London and was working with British *Vogue* when I suffered a jarring health crisis. I had a misdiagnosed gangrenous appendicitis that required an emergency operation. It took four hours of surgery and three doctors to save my life. They had to remove about 16 inches (40 centimeters) of my bowel, and it has taken me almost five years to fully recover. During this time, I learned a lot about nutrition's role in healing your body.

After two years of hard work, we are proud to bring you a compilation of healthy tips and recipes from around the world. We hope you enjoy the recipes and that our book leaves you *Good to Glow*!

Steph Adams

TALI'S PRINCIPLES

I believe in using simple ingredients in their most natural state. When I said I really cleaned up my diet, it meant saying goodbye to gluten, wheat germ, refined sugar, and genetically modified oils, as they can all be addictive, acidic, energy depleting, and difficult to digest.

No Gluten

Gluten is a protein found in wheat, barley, and rye. When flour is mixed with water, it produces a sticky, elastic protein that is known as gluten. The reason we avoid gluten is that this protein can cause inflammation in the gut and oxidation of the cells. When this happens, the body is unable to digest food efficiently and nutrients can't be properly absorbed. It can also cause bloating, tiredness, and congestion.

No Wheat Germ

Wheat germ also irritates the gut and is tied to many digestive issues. It can cause bacteria overgrowth and also affect the insulin levels in the body. Correct insulin levels are necessary to maintain healthy weight and energy levels.

No Refined Sugar

Refined sugar is considered by many experts to be a poison to the body, yet people consume it freely on a daily basis. It's a pure refined carbohydrate with no nutrient or mineral value. Instead, it causes premature aging by depleting collagen in the skin, leads to weight gain, and is highly addictive. Instead of using refined sugar, I use healthier natural substitutes such as xylitol, maple syrup, coconut sugar, rice syrup, and dates.

Good Fats and Oils

I don't believe in avoiding fats, but it is important to replace bad fats with the good ones that are necessary for the body and brain to function. I use coconut oil, olive oil, flaxseed oil, and avoid trans-fats and saturated fats. I also believe in eating healthy omega-3 fats available in wild-caught salmon and seeds. Omega-3 fats are essential for healthy hair, skin, and nails, not to mention weight control and emotional health.

STEPH'S TIPS

Drink 2 Liters of Water Every Day

Water helps flush your system of toxins, reduce stress, aid digestion, and help with weight loss. If you are exercising and eating well but not drinking enough water, you won't lose the weight as effectively.

Bathe in Epsom Salts

An epsom salt bath has been known to relieve inflammation, soothe aching pains, and treat migraine headaches. The magnesium in the epsom salts also help to produce serotonin and increase levels of adrenalin making you look better, feel better, and have more energy.

Follow the 80/20 Rule

I'd like to stay healthy 100% of the time, but it would be unrealistic to do this. I follow a healthy diet 80% of the time and allow myself whatever I feel like the other 20%. I always say that weekends are for enjoying yourself, but remember, it's all about balance.

Drink a Green Juice Every Day

Not only does it make you feel amazing, but having a green juice every day will help reduce skin cell damage thanks to its high antioxidant level.

Exercise Three Times a Week

It depends on how fit you are, but most people only need three sweat sessions a week to maintain a healthy body shape.

Use Detoxing Oils

Different natural oils contribute to different positive effects. To encourage the body to detox, try geranium, lavender, rosemary, and juniper oils. For relieving headaches, reach for rosemary, peppermint, and lavender. To relieve stress, use sandalwood, rose, or ylang-ylang. If you want to stimulate circulation, apply rose, thyme, juniper, and cypress. For a sleep aid, go with lavender, chamomile, clary sage, camphor, and rose.

10 WAYS TO MAKE YOUR SKIN GLOW

The key to glowing skin is not only what creams you rub on your face, but also what you eat. A balanced diet helps you stay fit, and it also makes sure that your skin stays healthy and radiant. Though you should eat everything in moderation, there are certain food items that help with glowing skin. Making them a part of your diet can do wonders for your complexion.

Water

Everyone can agree that good hydration keeps skin looking youthful and healthy. Shoot for drinking at least 1–2 liters of water a day. Choose pure, clean water, not liquids like soda and soup.

Carrots

For a powerful wrinkle-fighting boost, reach for carrots. This anti-aging vegetable is high in vitamin C, vitamin A, and beta-carotene that your skin needs to look great.

Berries

Berries—especially blueberries—are packed with antioxidants that neutralize damaging toxins in the body. They also help the body make collagen to keep your skin soft and smooth.

Green Tea

Green tea is so good for you, you'll want to fill up a big thermos of it in the morning and drink it all day long. Green tea is filled with antioxidants and anti-inflammatory properties.

Citrus

High in vitamin C, citrus is a glow-friendly food to have on hand at all times. Press your own to get the most vitamins and minerals and keep your skin looking young and fresh.

Nuts

Nuts are rich in vitamin E—an important antioxidant for the skin—and protein, meaning that this snack will not only get you glowing but keep you full too. Reap all of the benefits nuts have to offer by eating them unsalted, raw, and with the skins still intact. It's easy to add this skin-friendly food to your diet through salads, cereals, and on their own.

Coconut Yogurt

Make coconut yogurt a staple in your daily diet to enrich your skin with healthy enzymes and natural oils. Coconut yogurt can lead to smaller pores, better skin texture, and even be applied directly to your skin and hair topically. Replace mayonnaise and salad dressing with it to enjoy the benefits even more often.

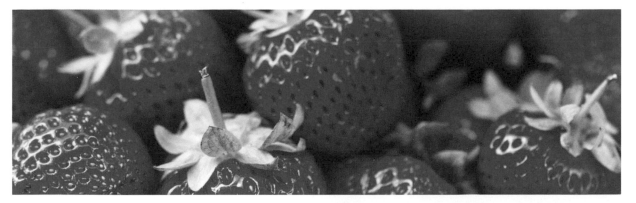

Sesame seeds

Sesame seeds add a crunchy kick to your diet and give your body boosts of vitamin E and copper to fight damage to the skin. Toss these seeds onto noodles, vegetables, curries, and in salads for a delicious dose of antioxidants.

Atlantic Salmon

With high levels of omega-3 fats that can help lower blood pressure, Atlantic salmon is a superfood worthy of eating at least two times per week.

Broccoli

Antioxidant-rich broccoli is a superfood must. It's filled with vitamin C, beta-carotene, and fiber.

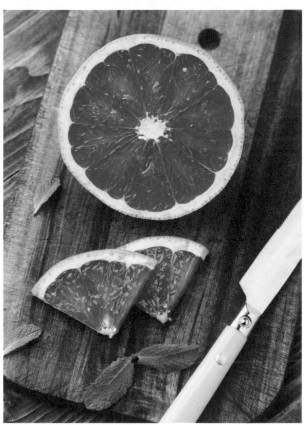

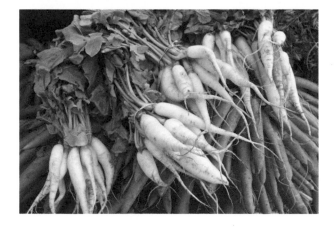

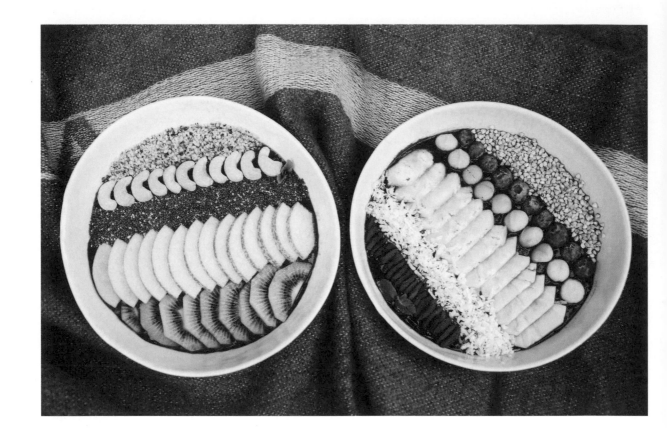

TOP SUPERFOODS

Quinoa

Quinoa is an anti-aging dream. The nutty grain is high in antioxidants while being low in calories (while still being filling!). This grain can act as an appetite suppressor thanks to its high protein content as well. Quinoa is great for those looking to shed some pounds!

Gluten-Free Oats

Slimmer waist anyone? Oats give your gut loads of filling fiber while lowering your body's bad cholesterol. This food keeps you full while helping your health, a great combination.

Pumpkin

Pumpkin packs a serious punch for healthy, glowing skin. It has nutrients like beta-carotene that rejuvenate skin, keep your eyes young, and aid aging bones.

Beans

For a vegetarian protein source, cook up some beans. This superfood brings together a perfect marriage of protein and fiber to keep your blood sugar from spiking after a meal and stabilize your mood. Satisfaction guaranteed!

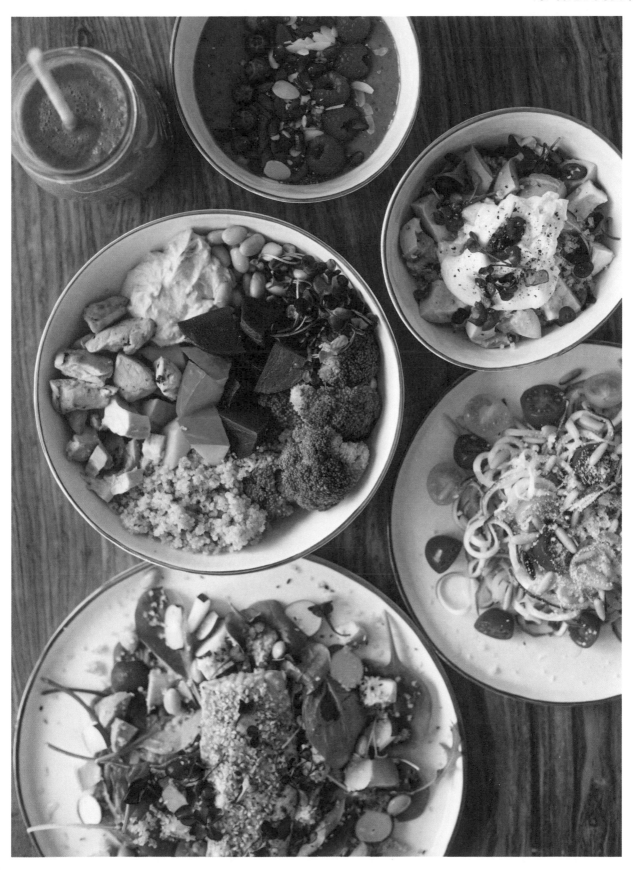

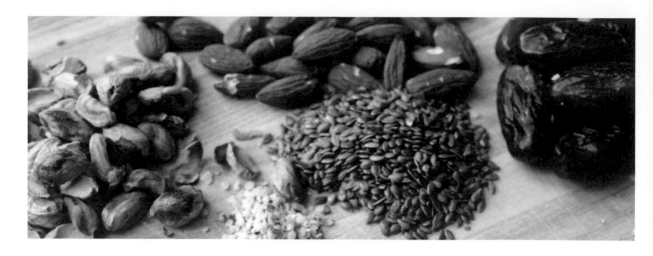

HOW TO MAKE SURE
YOU ARE GOOD TO GLOW

In the last few years, medical researchers worldwide have spoken about the benefits of alkalizing the body. This means that the pH levels of your body are more alkaline than acidic. When your body reaches the ideal balance of alkalinity and acidity, radiant good health is maximized and the result is vibrant skin that glows. This correct alkaline balance will help you feel light and bright, remove toxins, and shed unnecessary weight that may have built up over time.

The key to achieving the alkaline/acid balance is to reduce your stress level and consume less processed food, sugar, alcohol, dairy, and gluten (which are all acidic). The aim that we have with this book is to provide healthy and nutritious recipes that will help you increase the amount of alkalizing ingredients in your life. These include dark, leafy green vegetables such as kale, spinach, Swiss chard, parsley, and broccoli as well as high-quality oils like coconut oil and flaxseed oil. We had a lot of fun creating, compiling, and testing all of these recipes and we hope you love them!

Here are some of our other tips and principles that we have incorporated into our lives to help create the glow.

Hydration is Key

+ Drinking the correct amount of purified water is vital to create that glow. Drink at least 8 glasses of filtered water a day (never, ever tap) and add an extra glass of water for any coffee or black tea that you drink (if you really need to have coffee or black tea). We start the day drinking hot water with lemon and if we need to drink caffeine, then we make sure it is antioxidant-rich green tea. We also love making our own invigorating ginger and lemon tea as well as detoxifying herbal teas like dandelion, fennel, fresh mint, licorice, and chamomile before bed. Who said water has to be boring?

+ We always add 2 tablespoons of chlorophyll to filtered water at least once a day. Chlorophyll is amazing for detoxification and contains plenty of phytonutrients. You can find it in most pharmacies and health food stores.

Stress Busters

+ Massage is a great way to take time out for yourself, reduce stress, and get the lymphatic system working.

+ Increase exercise to help your body use oxygen and remove toxins through your lymphatic system. Exercise raises endorphins that create a healthy glow, and tones your body. We love daily brisk walks, yoga, and pilates.

+ Meditation and positive mantras are fantastic ways to make sure you are in the best frame of mind to glow from within. It may be cliché, but we believe that saying "What you think you become, what you feel you attract, what you imagine you create." It's true, so think healthy, happy, glowing thoughts!

Diet is Crucial

Alongside the delicious recipes in the book:

+ Try to eat seasonal produce. This means your produce is fresh and won't need nasty chemical preservatives.

+ Eat produce that is as close to its original form as possible.

+ Replace gluten with unrefined grains.

+ Eat organic ingredients.

+ While we try to get as many nutrients through food as possible, we also recommend seeing a professional nutritionist to advise on additional vitamin and mineral supplements you may need.

With these tips in mind, you are *Good to Glow*!

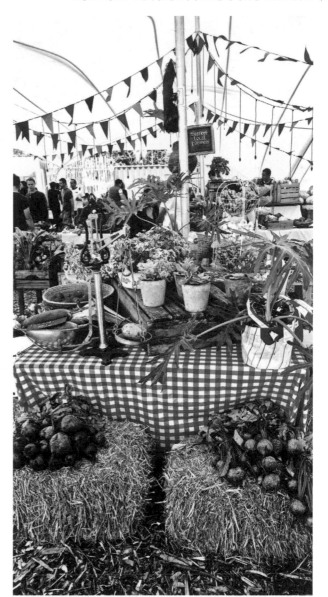

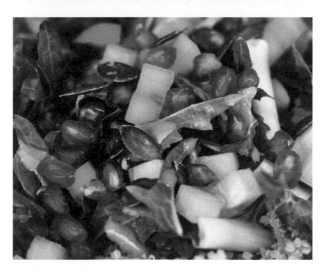

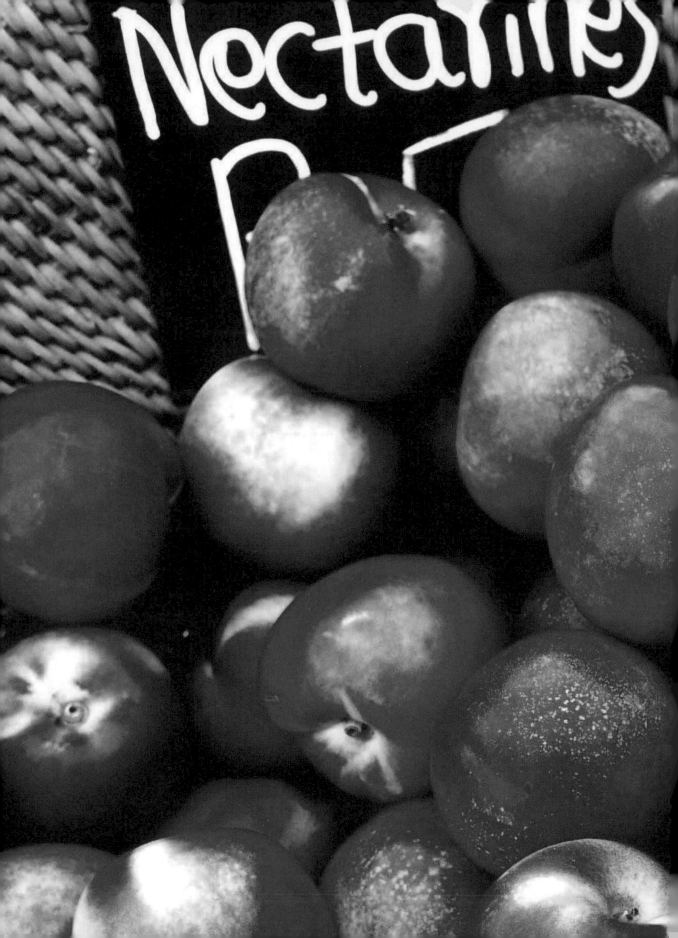

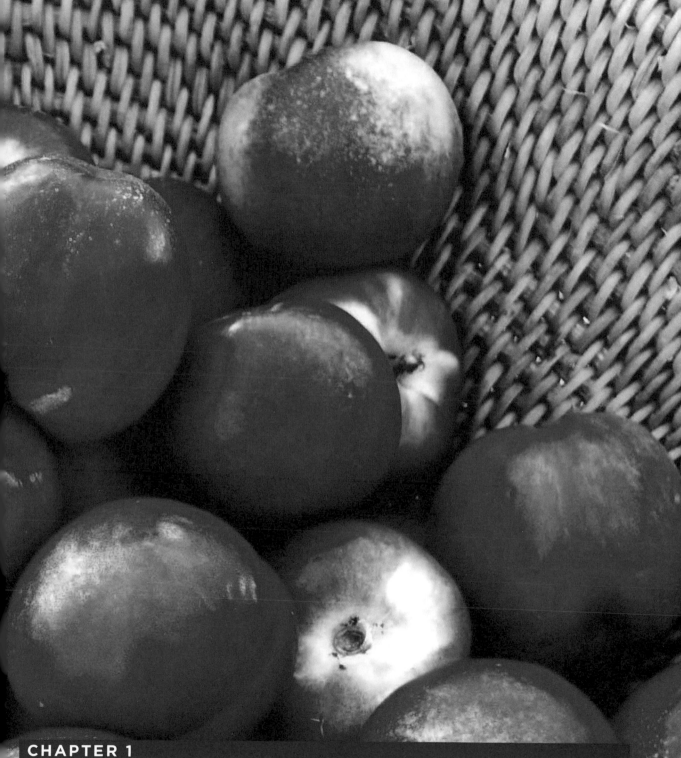

CHAPTER 1

JUICES & SMOOTHIES

LET'S GET JUICY

*Nothing will help your skin glow
more than a fresh juice or
blended smoothie.
These recipes contain some of
the most effective vegetables and
fruits for healing your body
and creating supple, beautiful,
radiant skin.*

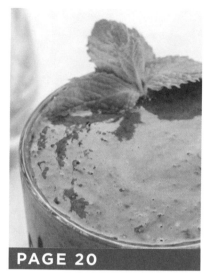

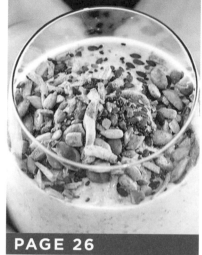

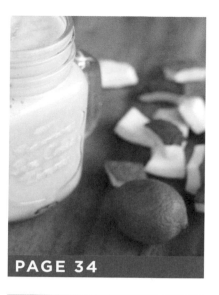

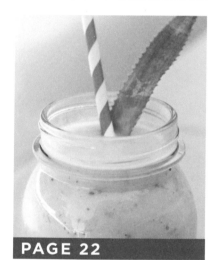

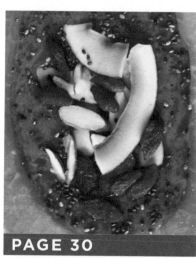

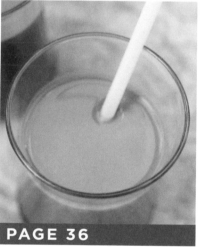

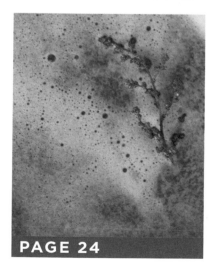

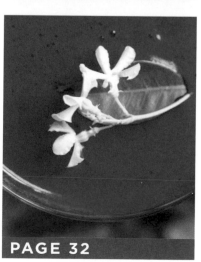

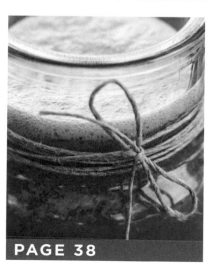

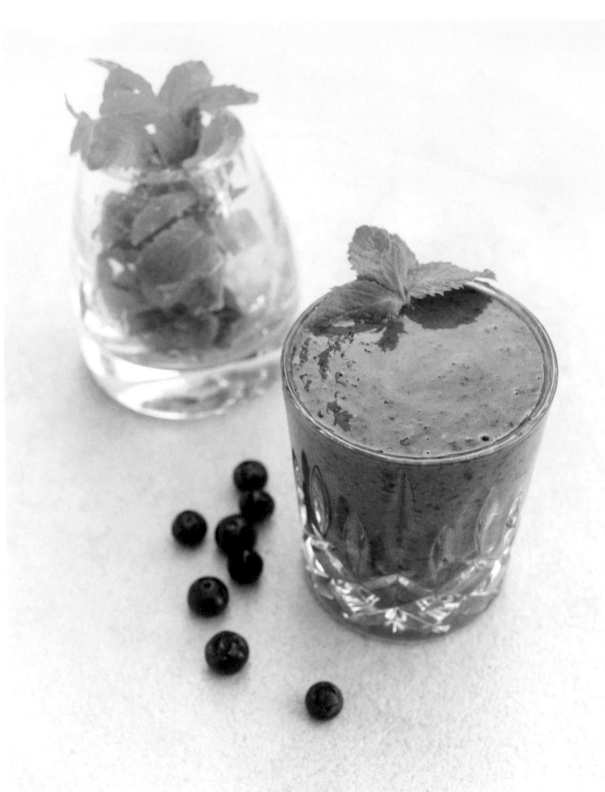

ELLE MACPHERSON
ANTI-OX BERRY BLITZER

PREPARATION

1) Wash berries and baby spinach leaves.

2) Blitz all ingredients in a blender until smooth.

3) Garnish with fresh berries.

INGREDIENTS

» *1 cup / 240 ml coconut water*
» *1 cup / 130 g fresh or frozen blueberries, or a mix of blueberries and raspberries*
» *1 cup / 30 g baby spinach leaves*
» *1 tbsp chia seeds*
» *2 tsp The Super Elixir by WelleCo*
» *Fresh berries for garnish*

ELLE MACPHERSON

Supermodel Elle Macpherson, otherwise known as "The Body," has carved out a diverse and purposeful career over the past 30 years. A prominent figure in business, fashion, film, and television, Elle has always undertaken endeavors with people and products that resonate with her values. Elle has recently co-founded WelleCo, a company dedicated to providing customers with the world's best whole food supplements as a way to improve nutrition and well-being.

www.ellemacpherson.com
www.welleco.com.au

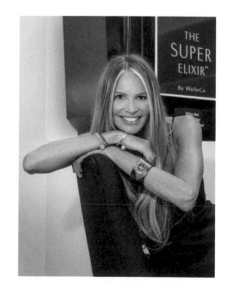

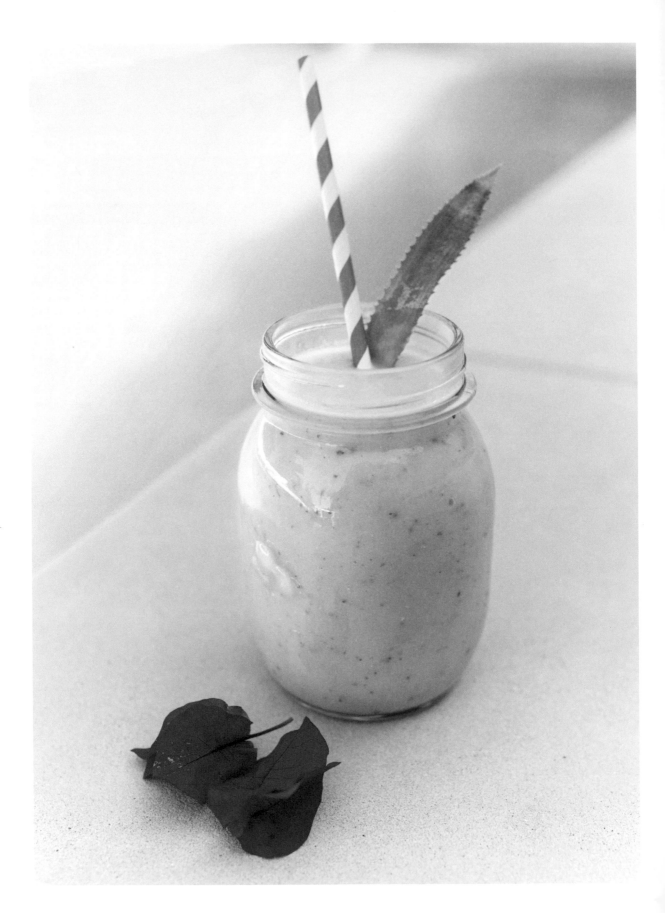

ELLE MACPHERSON
PIÑA COLADA SMOOTHIE

PREPARATION

1) Blitz all ingredients in your blender until smooth.

2) Serve immediately with a garnish of goji berries, coconut flakes, or fresh pineapple chunks.

INGREDIENTS

» *1 cup / 240 ml coconut water*
» *½ cup / 90 g pineapple chunks*
» *¼ avocado*
» *1 tbsp chia seeds*
» *2 tsp The Super Elixir by WelleCo*
» *1 tbsp lemon juice*
» *Some goji berries, coconut flakes, or fresh pineapple chunks for garnish*

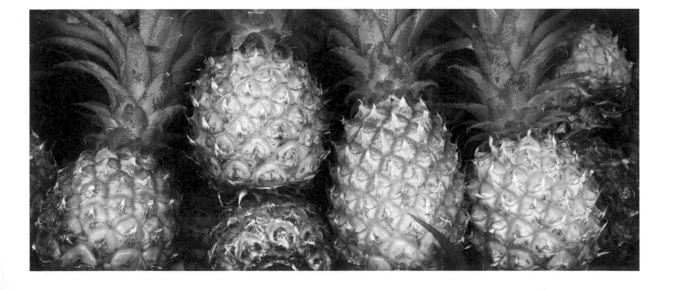

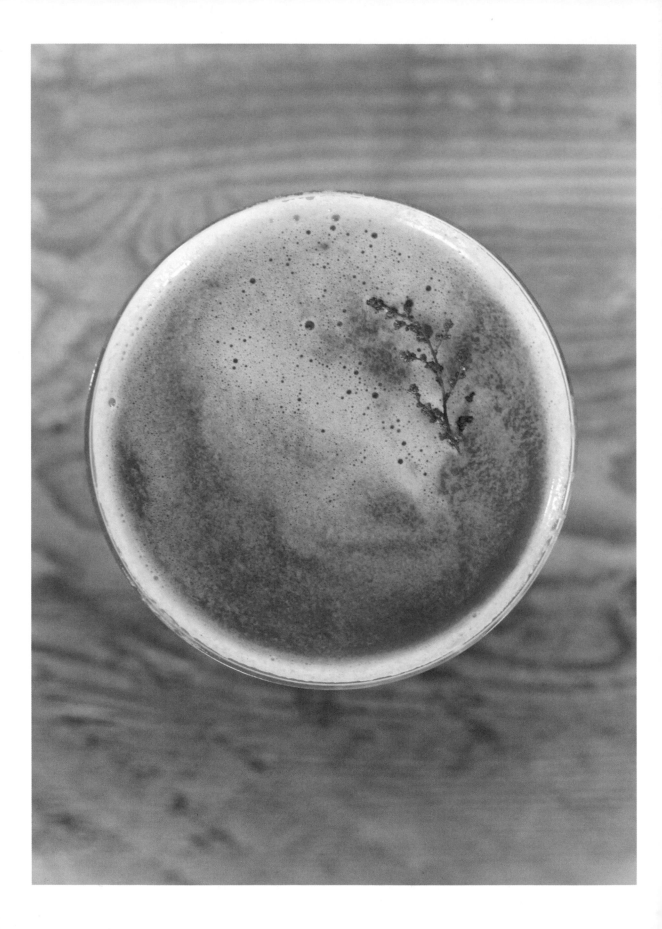

PLENISH CLEANSE
SUPERGREEN JUICE

PREPARATION

1) Wash all ingredients thoroughly.

2) Run all ingredients through your juicer.

3) Drink immediately and toast to your health!

INGREDIENTS

» *2 large cucumbers (peeled)*
» *1 large fistful of kale*
» *1 large fistful of sweet pea sprouts*
» *4–5 celery stalks*
» *1–2 broccoli stems*
» *1 pear or green apple*
» *Thumb-sized piece ginger (peeled)*

PLENISH CLEANSE

Founder of Plenish, Kara Rosen spent more than a decade at Condé Nast in New York working for magazines such as *Men's Vogue, Condé Nast Traveler,* and *People.* After a yearly battle against reoccurring strep throat and failing antibiotics, she turned to a holistic nutritionist who suggested a 5-day juice cleanse to get rid of the toxins that were attracting the strep. Skeptical, and worried about being hungry, Kara took a leap of faith. That 5-day cleanse—which began as temporary solution for an exhausted body—turned into a love for a new lifestyle. Kara began working with a talented nutritionist and created the right balance of phytonutrients and protein with the aim of making organic, cold-pressed juices readily available to everyone.

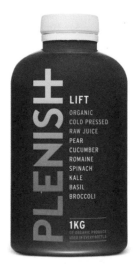

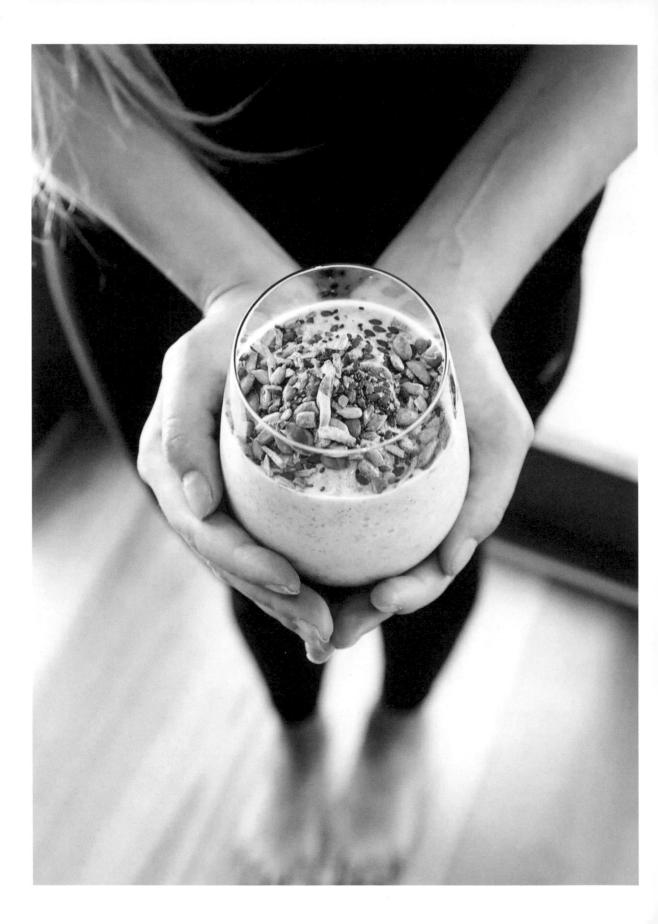

JESSICA SEPEL

CINNAMON, BANANA, & WALNUT SMOOTHIE

PREPARATION

1) Place all the ingredients into a blender and mix all together until you reach a smooth consistency.

2) Garnish smoothie with crushed nuts, seeds, or gluten-free muesli.

INGREDIENTS

» *1 serving vanilla whey protein powder or 2 tbsp ground flaxseed-sunflower-almond mix*
» *1 tbsp Greek yogurt (optional)*
» *2 tbsp raw walnuts*
» *¼ or ½ ripe banana (frozen banana works as well)*
» *1 tbsp pumpkin seeds*
» *1 tsp stevia/maple syrup*
» *1 tsp cinnamon*
» *½ tsp nutmeg*
» *1 tsp vanilla powder*
» *Squeeze of lemon*
» *1 cup / 140 g ice*
» *1 cup / 240 ml sugar-free almond milk*
» *Crushed nuts, seeds, gluten-free muesli for garnish*

JESSICA SEPEL

Jessica Sepel is a nutritionist and the author of *The Healthy Life*. With a degree in health science and an advanced diploma in nutritional medicine, Jessica has an approach to healthy living informed by a well-researched understanding of nutrition, complimented by a passion to achieve a physical and psychological balance. She is driven to help individuals embrace a healthier lifestyle through diet and believes food can heal all.

www.jessicasepel.com

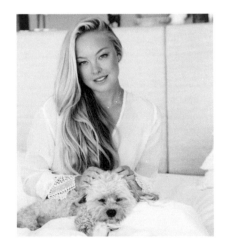

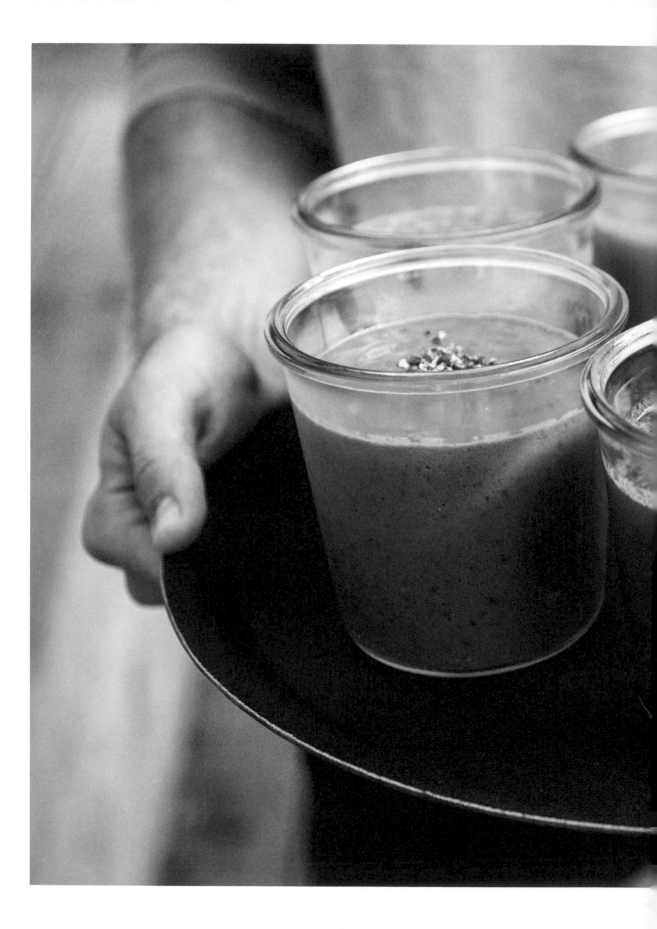

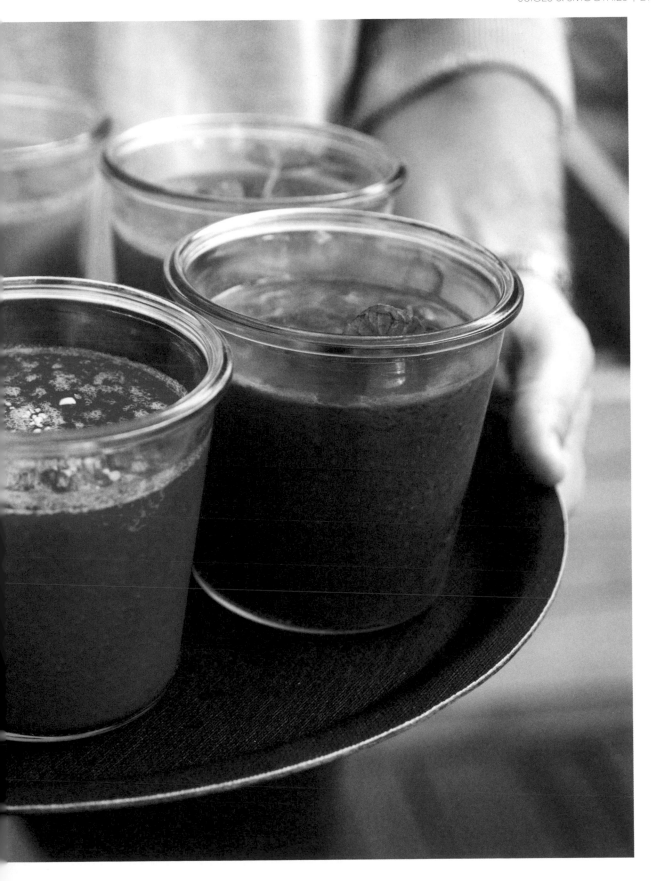

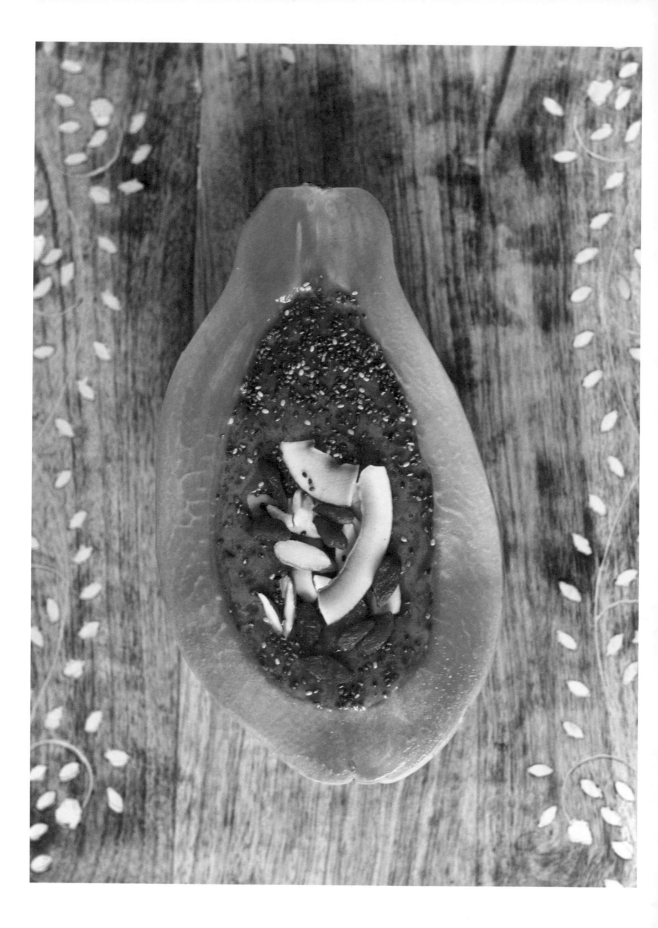

JULIE STEVANJA
BERRY SMOOTHIE

PREPARATION

1) In a high-speed blender, blend coconut water with the frozen banana, berries, and a scoop of Bare Blends Protein Powder.

2) Pour it into a bowl or fill the hollow of a papaya.

3) Garnish with goji berries, slivered almonds, chia seeds, and toasted coconut.

INGREDIENTS

» *1 cup / 240 ml coconut water*
» *½ frozen banana*
» *½ cup / 65 g raspberries*
» *¼ cup / 30 g blueberries*
» *1 scoop of Bare Blends Protein Powder*

Garnish:
» *Goji berries*
» *Slivered almonds*
» *Chia seeds*
» *Coconut (toasted)*
» *½ papaya (deseeded) (optional)*

JULIE STEVANJA

In 2012, Julie Stevanja co-founded and launched Stylerunner.com, one of the world's first activewear e-commerce sites to curate pieces from top sportswear brands including Nike, Adidas, Reebok, Puma, and lululemon athletica. Today, the CEO is also a keynote speaker and regularly recognized for her involvement in Australia's startup landscape.

www.stylerunner.com

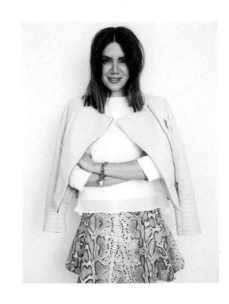

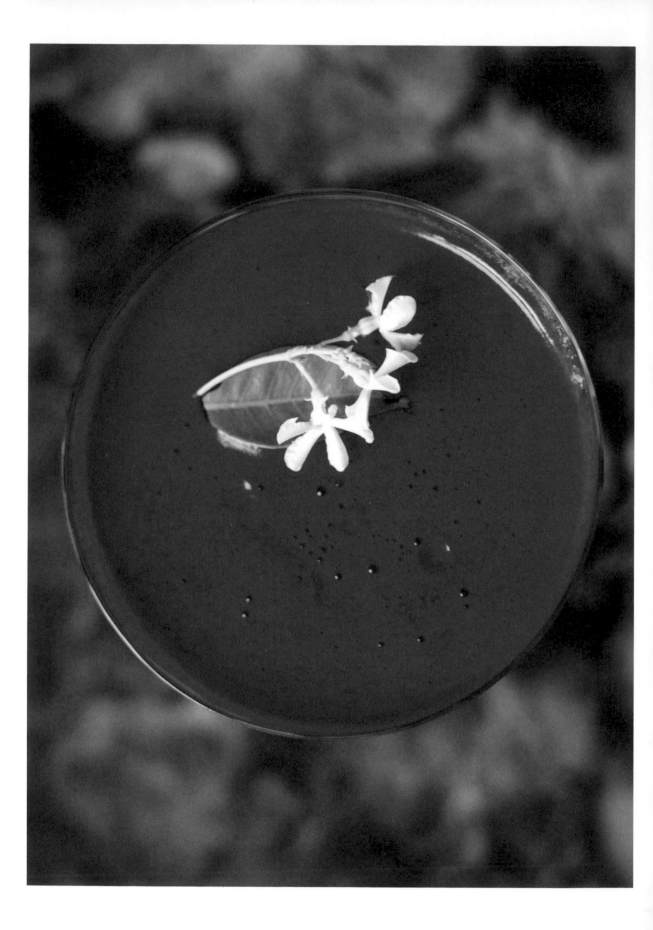

SOUTH KENSINGTON CLUB
SUPER BEET JUICE

PREPARATION

1) Wash all ingredients thoroughly.

2) Add all ingredients into your blender and mix well.

INGREDIENTS

» *6 medium beets (peeled)*
» *1 medium red apple*
» *3 tbsp lemon juice*
» *4 large carrots (peeled)*
» *Thumb-sized piece ginger (peeled)*

SOUTH KENSINGTON CLUB

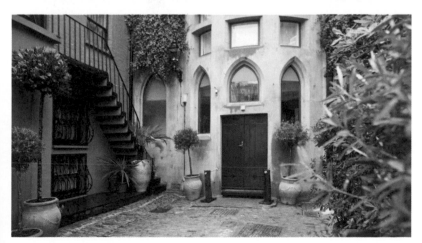

London's newest members club, South Kensington Club is based in the heart of prestigious South Kensington. The private club offers a state-of-the-art gymnasium, spa, library, juice bar, Watsu pool, Turkish Hammam, and Russian Banya.

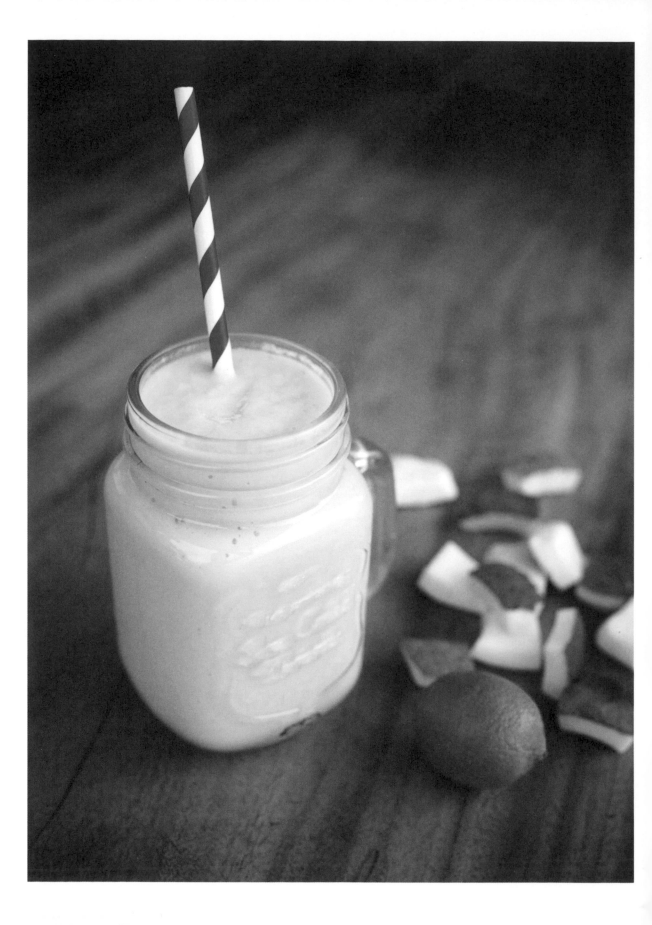

IMBIBERY LONDON
SUPER SMOOTHIE

PREPARATION

1) Wash all ingredients thoroughly.

2) Add all ingredients into your blender and mix well.

Good to Know:
The combination of baobab, avocado, and mango
is great for your skin, helping you keep that summer glow
all year round.

INGREDIENTS

» ¼ avocado
» ¼ mango (diced)
» ¼ cup / 60 ml lime juice
  (add more or less depending on
  how much of a kick you want)
» ½ cup / 120 ml coconut water
» ½ cup / 120 ml filtered water
» 1 tsp baobab powder

IMBIBERY LONDON

Imbibery London's mission is to make juice work for everyone.
The cold-pressed juice brand believes its nutrient-rich juice
will consume you entirely, giving its products names like
the Intoxicating Detox and the Goddess Cleanse. Imbibery believes
that those who "imbibe" live life to the fullest; they're empowered
to jet and reset when they incorporate raw, unpasteurized,
cold-pressed juice into their everyday routine.

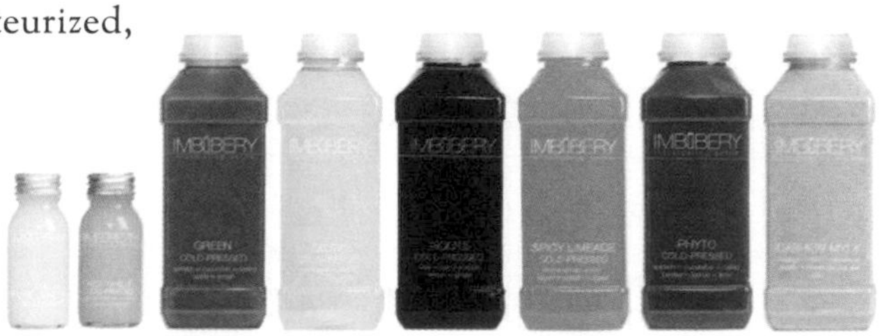

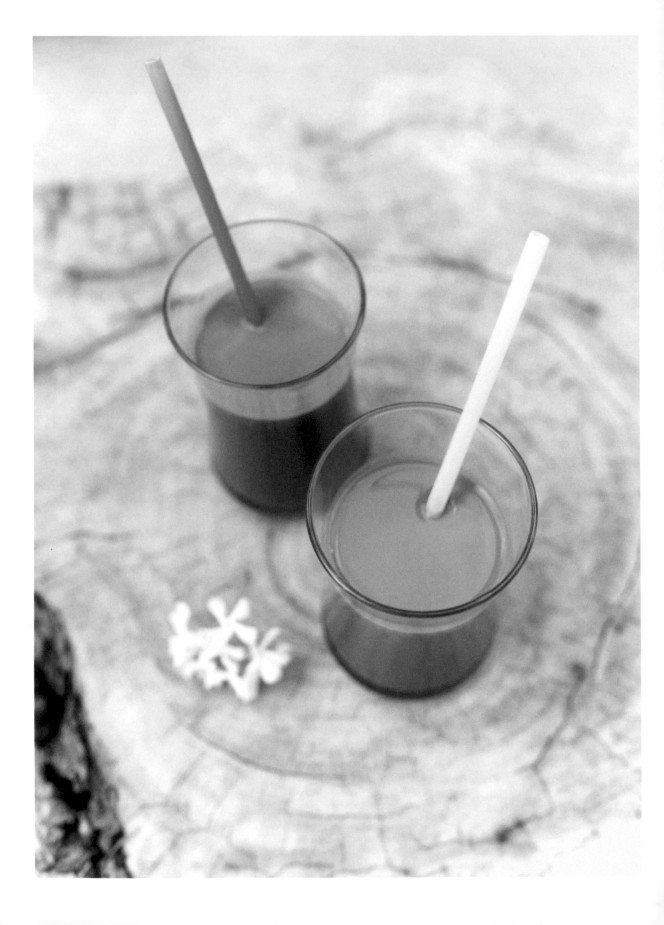

CRUDE JUICE
CHOCO MACA MYLK

PREPARATION

1) Place all ingredients (except the cacao nibs) into your blender. Blend until thick and frothy.

2) Add in the handful of cacao nibs and blend on slow for 20 seconds. The idea is to have a bit of crunch at the end.

INGREDIENTS

(Serves 2)

- » *4 ⅕ cups / 1 l filtered water*
- » *1 ⅕ cups / 150 g cashews*
- » *1 handful of dates*
- » *1 tbsp maca powder*
- » *2 tbsp raw cacao powder*
- » *1 tbsp lucuma powder*
- » *Pinch of sea salt*
- » *1 vanilla bean (seeds only)*
- » *1 handful of cacao nibs*

CRUDE JUICE

The idea to launch Crude came when founder Guy Robinson was in New York working as a model. Working in the fashion industry acted as a precursor to leading a healthy and balanced lifestyle. Juicing just seemed to fit perfectly into a hectic traveling and work schedule. He juiced regularly to keep his energy levels topped up and began experiencing firsthand how amazing liquid nutrition could be. He was in awe as the cold-pressed juice movement gathered speed in New York. When he returned to London, Guy was unable to find the cold-pressed juice that he was used to, so he set up his own company and threw his passion behind it.

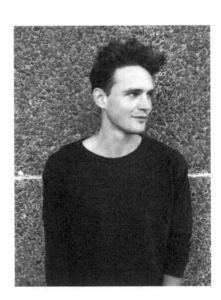

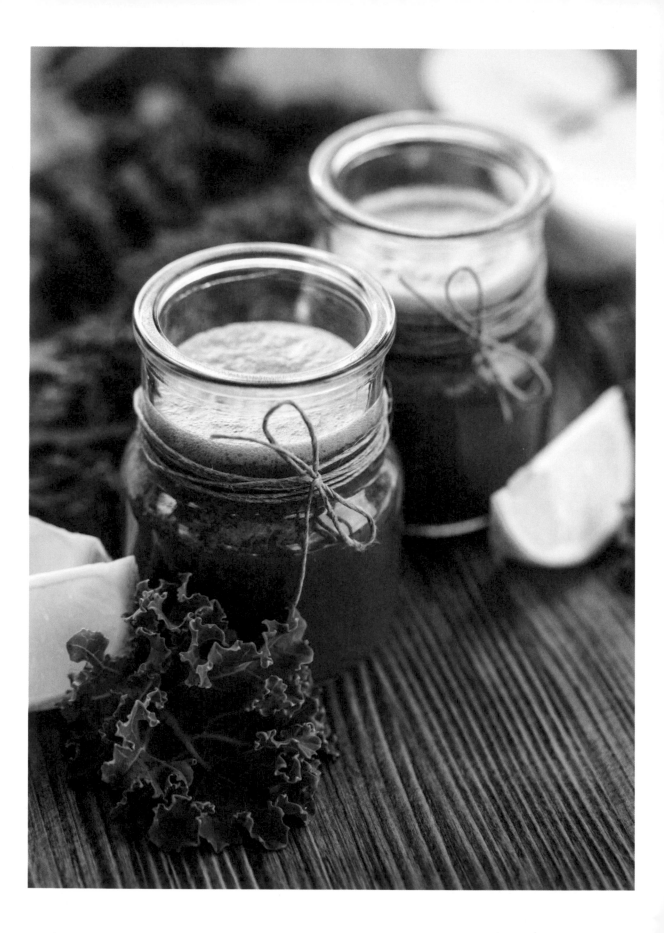

STEPH ADAMS
SUPER GREEN SMOOTHIE

PREPARATION

1) Blend all ingredients in high-powered blender.

2) Top with chia seeds and serve fresh.

INGREDIENTS

» *1 handful of spinach*
» *1 handful of kale*
» *1 frozen mango*
» *½ banana*
» *½ cup / 125 ml almond milk*
» *Filtered water to taste*
» *Spirulina (optional)*
» *Pinch of bee pollen and black chia seeds to garnish*

STEPH SAYS:

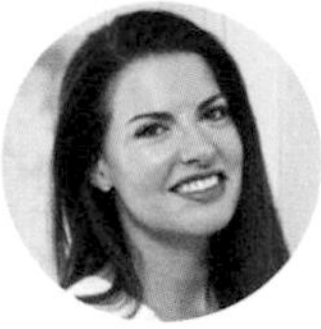

"This smoothie is so good for you and will keep your skin glowing. If you have trouble getting your daily amount of fruit and vegetables into your system, then this smoothie will have you good to glow!"

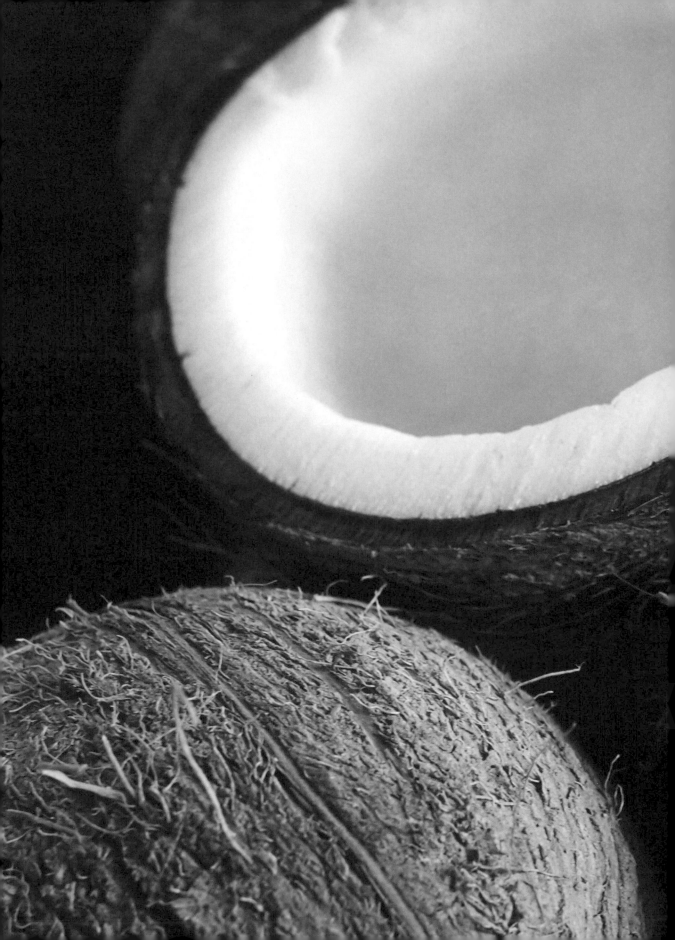

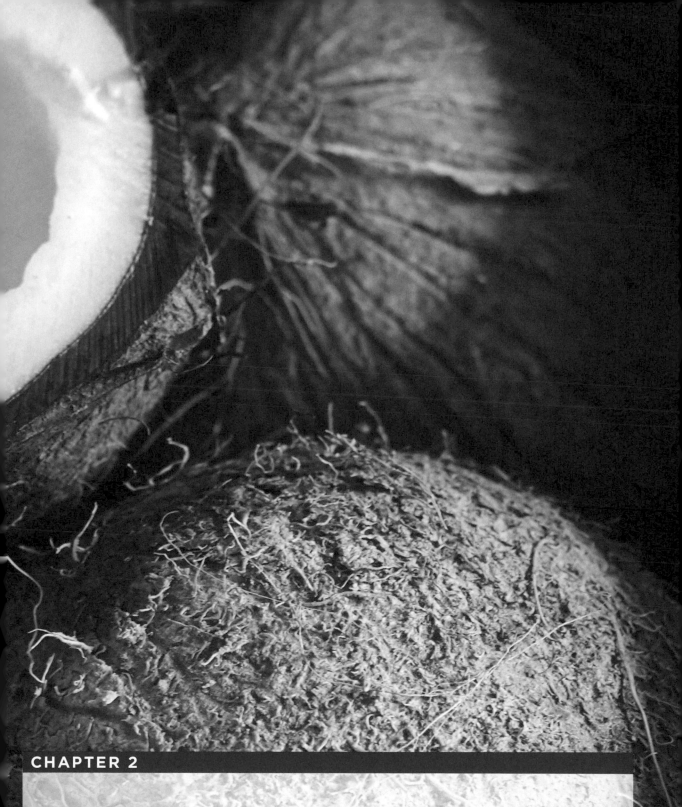

CHAPTER 2

BREAKFAST & BRUNCH

HAVE A BREAK

*These dishes can create
the perfect start to any day.
Whether you're having friends
over for a casual brunch up,
or bringing your family together
for a leisurely breakfast,
these recipes will make for
a wonderful morning menu.*

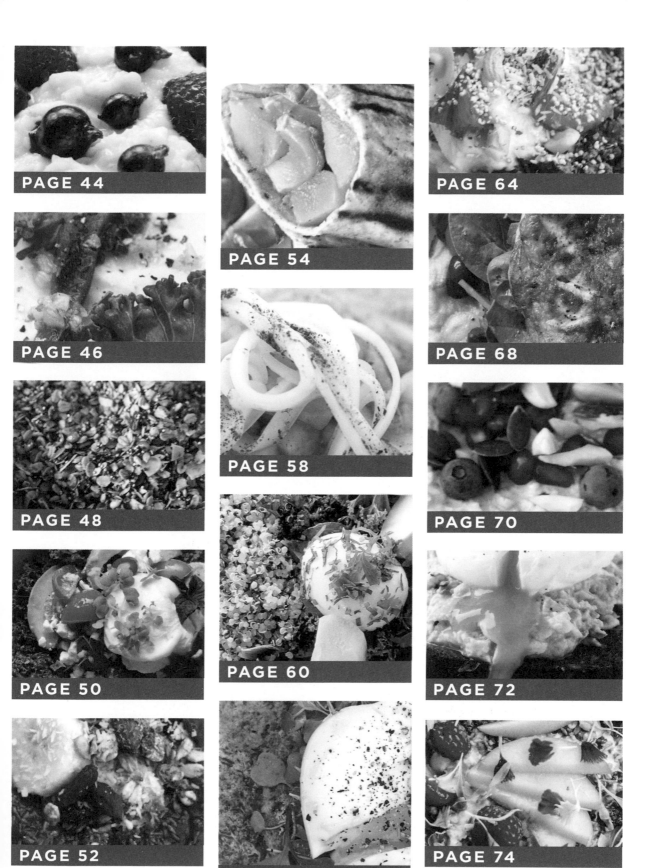

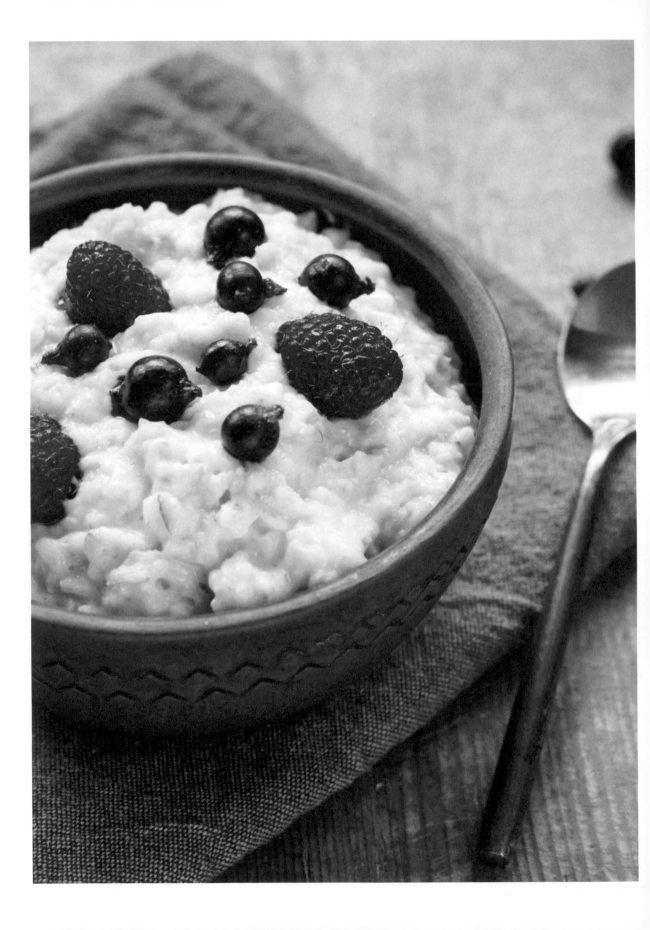

STEPH ADAMS

OATS WITH QUINOA & BLUEBERRIES

PREPARATION

1) Combine the oats and quinoa into a bowl.

2) Add your choice of almond milk or yogurt.

3) Garnish with fruit.

INGREDIENTS

» *1 cup / 90 g oats*
» *½ cup / 95 g quinoa flakes*
» *2 cups / 480 ml yogurt or almond milk*
» *¼ cup / 30 g blueberries*
» *3 raspberries*

STEPH SAYS:

"The quinoa in this dish keeps you full of energy all day."

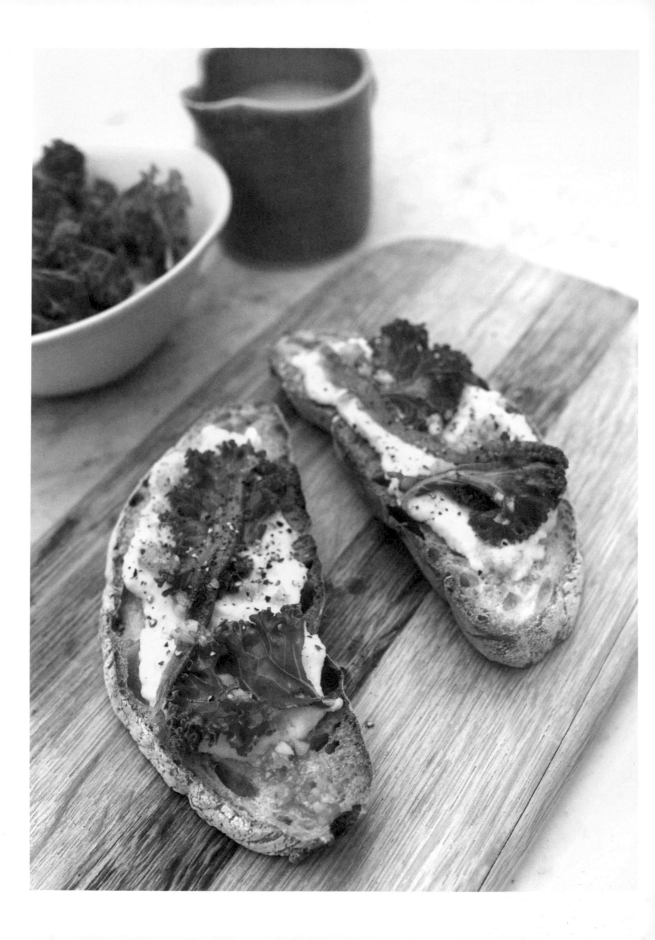

DE KAS
CAULIFLOWER & KALE CROSTINI

PREPARATION

Crème:
1) Preheat oven to 390°F / 200°C.
2) Wash the cauliflower, slice it into equal parts.
3) Put a small amount of water in the bottom of a baking dish with the thyme twigs.
4) Place the cauliflower in the dish and cover with aluminum foil.
5) Put in the oven for 20 minutes.
6) Check after 20 minutes to see if the cauliflower is cooked (it will be soft). Remove and blend with the olive oil to create a smooth crème.
7) Add salt to taste.

Crostini:
1) Slice the bread and cover with olive oil. Toast the bread on the grill or pan so it's crispy. Do not scorch the bread.
2) When the bread is toasted, scrape the clean clove of garlic over the surface.
3) Spread cauliflower crème over the top.
4) Portion the anchovy together with the kale over the crostini.
5) Finish with a little bit of salt, black pepper, a sprinkle of olive oil, and the gremolata.

INGREDIENTS

(Serves 4)

Crème:
- » *1 small cauliflower*
- » *½ cup / 110 g cold-pressed virgin olive oil*
- » *Sea salt to taste*
- » *2 twigs thyme*

Crostini:
- » *Fresh gluten-free or sourdough bread*
- » *1 clove fresh garlic*
- » *Extra-virgin olive oil to taste*
- » *Sea salt and black pepper to taste*
- » *For every crostino, 1 fillet salted anchovy (optional)*
- » *1 handful of blanched kale*
- » *Gremolata (finely chopped garlic, fried while slowly stirring, until golden brown)*

DE KAS

De Kas Restaurant and Nursery is dreamily situated in what was once the Amsterdam City Greenery. It's no surprise that De Kas was created with an ethos that food tastes best when it is prepared using the freshest ingredients, after all, it boasts its own greenhouses and garden near the restaurant where seasonal Mediterranean vegetables, herbs, and edible flowers are harvested with respect for nature.

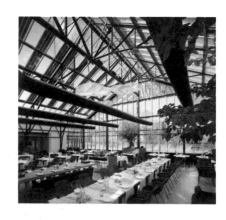

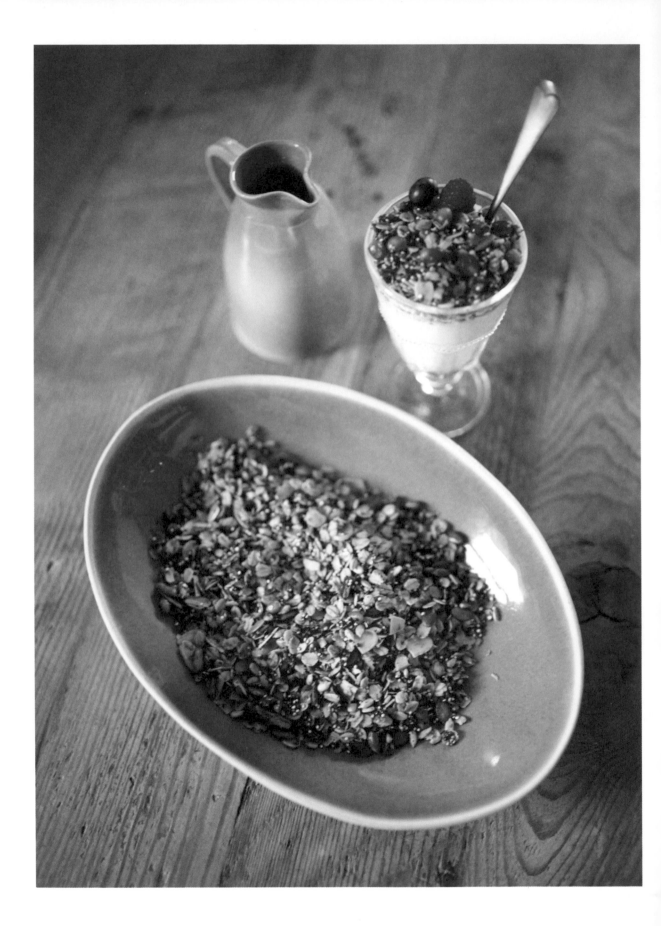

TALI SHINE
QUINOA GRANOLA

PREPARATION

1) Preheat oven to 350°F / 180°C.

2) Place all the dry ingredients into a bowl (quinoa, oats, seeds, cinnamon, and nuts), then add the wet ingredients (coconut oil and maple syrup). Mix thoroughly.

3) Grease a baking tray with coconut oil or line with baking paper.

4) Spread the mixture along the baking tray.

5) Bake for 15 minutes or until golden brown, turning over as necessary (the sliced almonds will brown fast!).

6) Serve with coconut yogurt, almond milk, berries, or seasonal fruit.

INGREDIENTS

- » 2 ⅓ cups / 400 g white quinoa
- » 4 ½ cups / 400 g gluten-free oats
- » ½ cup / 100 g pumpkin seeds
- » ¼ cup / 20 g sliced almonds
- » ¼ cup / 25 g pecans
- » ½ cup / 65 g sunflower seeds
- » 1 tbsp cinnamon
- » 3 tbsp coconut oil
- » 4 ½ tbsp maple syrup

TALI SAYS:

"This tasty granola is easy to make and filled with protein, omegas, and fiber. It is delicious on its own, as a snack, or with homemade almond milk, coconut yogurt, and berries."

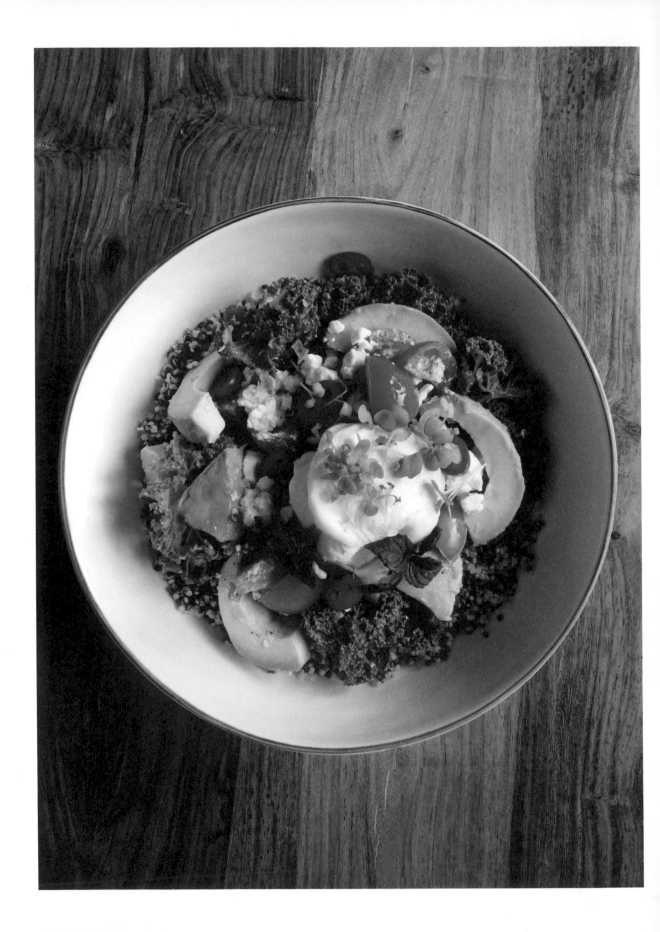

LAURA'S DELI
PROTEIN POWER EGG

PREPARATION

1) Cook all the ingredients for the vegetable stock with about 4 cups / 1 liter of water.
2) Use half of the stock to cook the quinoa for about 6–7 minutes and let sit for 2 more minutes.
3) Heat the coconut oil in a pan and steam the spring onion and cherry tomatoes.
4) Add the feta cheese until it melts lightly, then add cilantro and chili. Toss together in a pan for a short time.
5) Blanch kale in the second half of the stock for about 1 minute.
6) Put water with a little bit of vinegar in a small pot and bring to a simmer (don't boil). With a spoon, create a swirl in the middle of the pot and let egg (without the shell) fall into the swirl to poach. Cook for about 4 minutes.
7) Rinse cooked quinoa with cold water.
8) First put quinoa in a bowl, then make a nest of kale, then put hot tomatoes and feta on top of the kale.
9) Spread small avocado pieces into bowl.
10) Place poached egg into center. Salt and pepper to taste.

INGREDIENTS

Vegetable Stock:
  » *2 carrots*
  » *2 leeks*
  » *2 celery stalks*
  » *2 bay leaves*

Dish:
  » *1 ⅛ cups / 200 g quinoa*
  » *½ cup / 90 g feta cheese*
  » *1 spring onion (chopped)*
  » *Approximately 10 cherry tomatoes (quartered)*
  » *1 tbsp coconut oil*
  » *Fresh cilantro*
  » *1 fresh chili (chopped)*
  » *Approximately 4 big kale leaves*
  » *1 egg*
  » *½ to 1 ripe avocado (sliced)*
  » *Himalayan pink salt*
  » *Pepper*
  » *Vinegar*

LAURA'S DELI

Laura Koerver is the founder of the clean food restaurant Laura's Deli in Düsseldorf, Germany. After working in the fashion and marketing industry, she chose a new career direction and landed in the food world. She changed her own diet, worked in the kitchen of a raw food restaurant in London, and eventually implemented her own ideas and passion to open Laura's Deli. The menu is an interpretation of modern nutrition based on medical findings and international trends, offering a mix of innovative and nutrient-rich products served in a modern atmosphere.

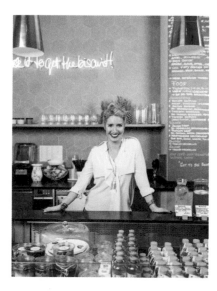

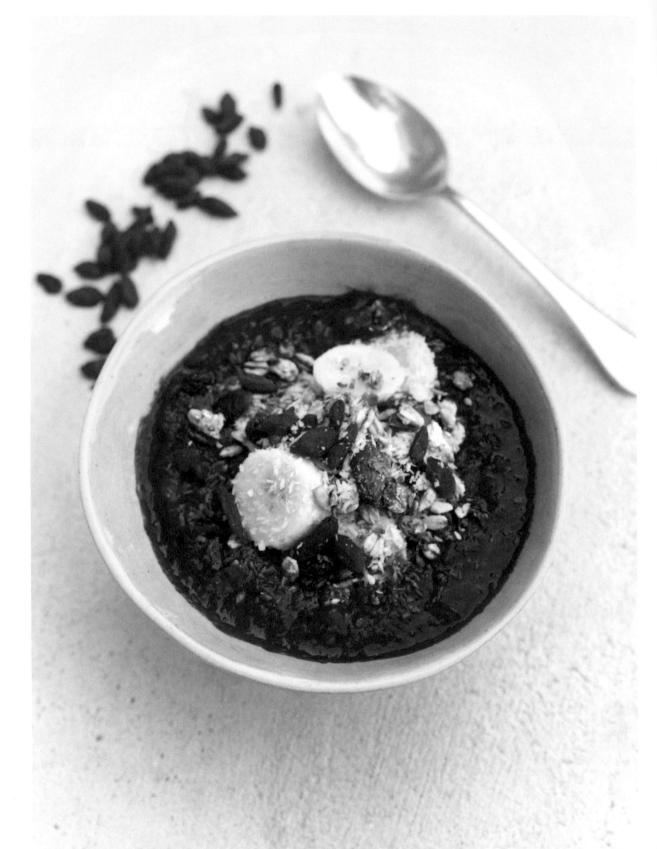

DEBORAH SYMOND
AÇAÍ BREAKFAST BOWL

PREPARATION

1) Combine açai, banana, strawberries, and apple juice (or almond/coconut milk). Blend until smooth.

2) Spoon into serving bowl(s) and garnish with bananas, blueberries, coconut, granola, and goji berries.

INGREDIENTS

» *2 tbsp açai berry powder*
» *1 banana (plus ½ cup / 115 g sliced bananas for garnish)*
» *1 cup / 150 g frozen strawberries*
» *½ cup / 120 g apple juice (replace with almond or coconut milk for a creamier consistency)*

Garnish:
» *⅓ cup / 45 g blueberries*
» *¼ cup / 25 g shredded coconut*
» *⅓ cup / 35 g granola (flaxseed, gluten-free, or regular sugar-free granola)*
» *¼ cup / 30 g goji berries*

DEBORAH SYMOND

Tastemaker Deborah Symond is the founder of the lifestyle site modesportif.com, an online destination dedicated to luxe sports leisurewear. She loves health and fitness and can be found doing spin, yoga, and TRX classes in the chicest outfits all around the world. Deborah is also a bonafide foodie who loves to cook and believes that healthy food should still be delicious.

www.modesportif.com

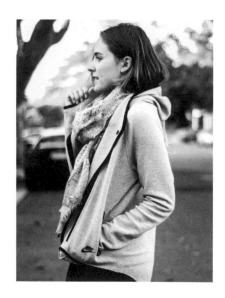

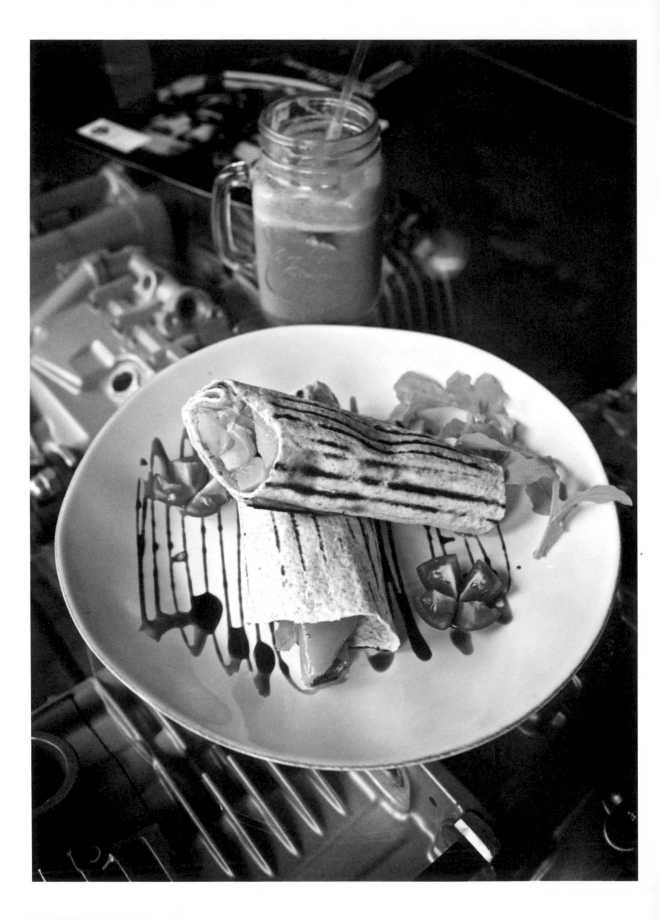

TRIBE 112 CAFÉ
THE VEG-VEG WRAP

PREPARATION

Wrap:
1) Mix flour, margarine, and 6–8 tablespoons of water together in a bowl until you have a rough dough. Cover the bowl with a towel and place in the fridge for 30 minutes. After that, knead dough again.
2) Divide the dough into 6 portions. Roll each portion nice and thin into about 7–8-in. / 20 cm circles and put them on a piece of floured wax paper.
3) Give them a sear for 1–2 minutes in a hot, dry pan (don't use any oil!). When they get puffy, use a fork to let the hot air out.
4) Serve immediately, or cool slightly before storing in a plastic bag.

Hummus:
1) Rinse chickpeas in cold water and place into your blender.
2) Add the tahini, crushed garlic, herbs, spices, and lemon juice (leave out the paprika and parsley). Turn on the blender and slowly pour in the oil.
3) When the mixture is fully combined and smooth, sprinkle with paprika and finely chopped parsley leaves for color.

Vegetable Filling:
1) Cut the bell pepper, red onion, and garlic into strips.
2) Roast onions and garlic in a frying pan with olive oil over high heat. Add bell peppers and cook over medium heat until the vegetables begin to soften.
3) Season with salt and pepper.

To Serve:
1) Spread some hummus over each wrap. Top with fresh salad and vegetable filling, then roll each of them up. Shortly before serving, heat wraps again in a frying pan or in the oven to enjoy warm.

INGREDIENTS

(For 2 wraps)

Wrap:
- *⅓ cup and 1 tbsp / 50 g gluten-free flour*
- *2 tsp vegetable margarine*
- *Pinch of salt*

Hummus:
- *1 cup / 180 g chickpeas (soaked overnight and well-cooked)*
- *1 tbsp tahini*
- *2 tbsp extra-virgin olive oil*
- *1 garlic clove (crushed)*
- *1 tbsp lemon juice*
- *Salt, ground cumin, and ground pepper to taste*
- *Paprika and fresh parsley leaves (chopped) for garnish*

Vegetable Filling:
- *1 yellow bell pepper*
- *1 green bell pepper*
- *½ red onion*
- *1 garlic clove*
- *Salt and ground pepper to taste*
- *Extra-virgin olive oil*
- *Fresh green salad for garnish*

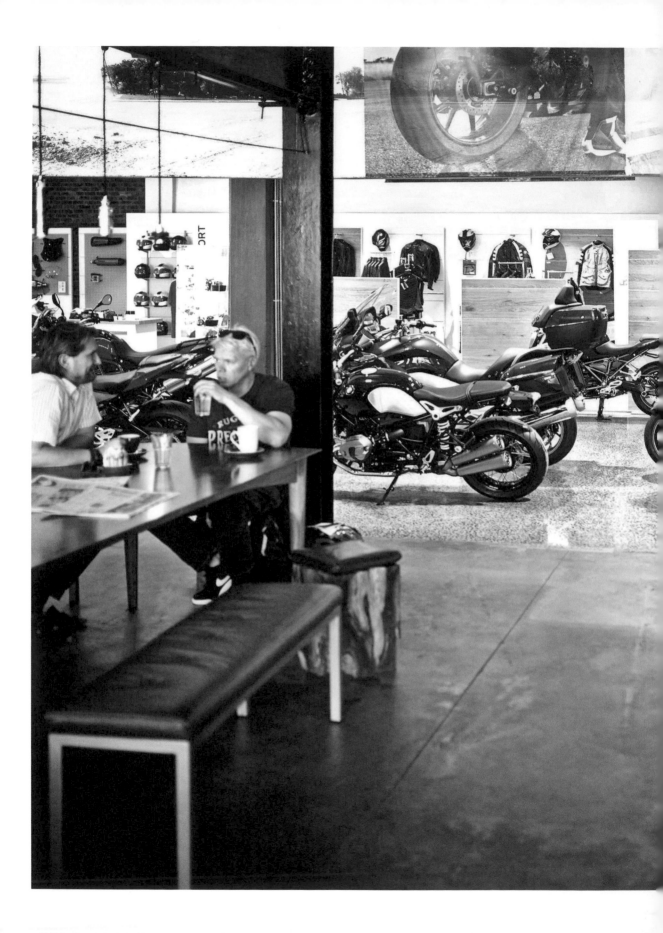

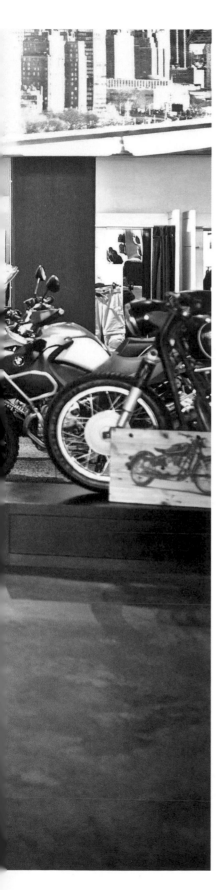

TRIBE 112 CAFÉ

With a mission to offer luxury coffee to everyone, Tribe Coffee is one of Cape Town's most respected roasters. At the brand's new concept Tribe 112 Café, craft coffee and motorcycle culture come together in a modern and elegant space. In addition to decadent dishes like Traditional Bacon and Eggs, the café serves diet-friendly foods like the Bircher Oats Bowl and this Veg-Veg Wrap.

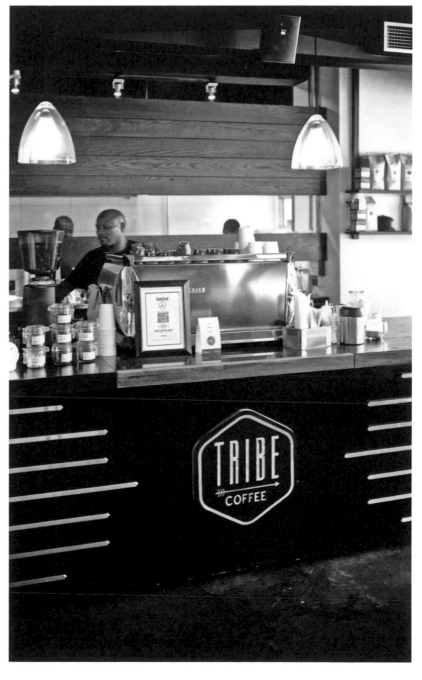

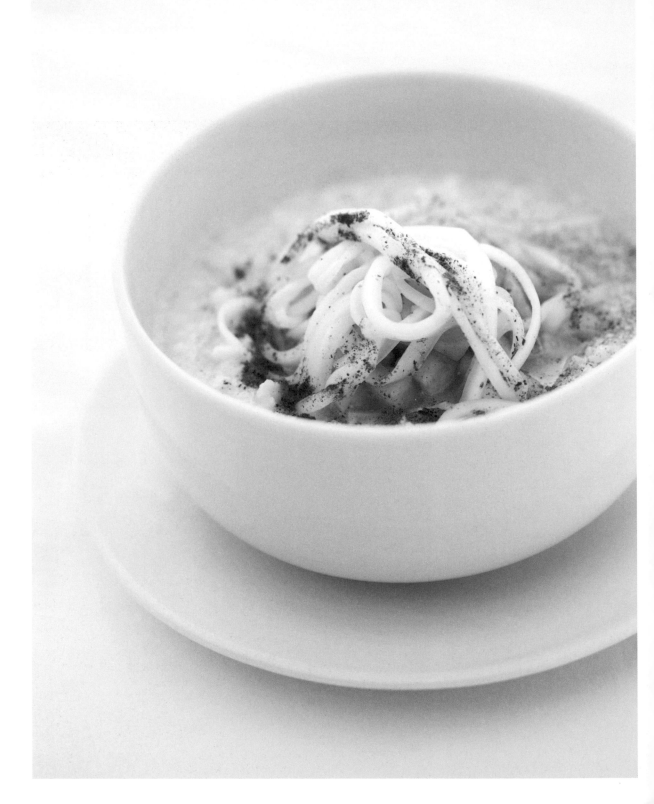

COMO SHAMBHALA ESTATE
CINNAMON PORRIDGE

PREPARATION

Coconut water is lauded for its low-calorie, high-electrolyte properties, while coconut meat can help improve the body's immune system and anti-inflammatory responses. Achieving a porridge-like consistency is all about how you blend the young coconut meat and water with the almonds. It needs to be done on the lowest speed; if blended too quickly, it will end up as a purée.

1) Place the almonds in a bowl, cover with water and soak for 12 hours.
2) Drain and rinse the almonds, then place them in a blender with the coconut water. Using the pulse button, blend until the nuts are coarsely chopped.
3) Add the coconut meat, coconut or agave nectar, vanilla seeds, and sea salt. Pulse until you have a coarse consistency.

Spiced Coconut Water:
1) Combine coconut water with ground cinnamon and coconut or agave nectar, mixing well.
2) Cover and refrigerate until ready to serve.

To serve:
1) Combine the coconut meat with the fruit.
2) Drizzle with spiced coconut water and toss gently to combine.
3) Spoon the porridge into chilled bowls and top with the dressed fruit.
4) Finish with a sprinkling of cinnamon.

INGREDIENTS

(Serves 4)

Porridge:
  » *3 cups / 320 g flaked almonds*
  » *½ cup / 120 ml young coconut water*
  » *2 cups / 300 g young coconut meat*
  » *1 tbsp coconut or agave nectar*
  » *½ vanilla bean, split lengthwise*
  » *Pinch of sea salt*

Spiced Coconut Water:
  » *½ cup / 120 ml young coconut water*
  » *Pinch of cinnamon*
  » *1 tbsp coconut or agave nectar*

Garnish:
  » *¼ cup / 35 g young coconut meat (julienned)*
  » *¼ cup / 35 g red papaya (diced)*
  » *1 banana (peeled, thinly sliced)*
  » *8 strawberries (quartered)*
  » *2 pinches of cinnamon*

COMO SHAMBHALA ESTATE

The COMO resorts around the world are renowned for their chic design and fantastic dining programs. At COMO Shambhala Estate's restaurant Glow in stunning Bali, Indonesia, guests have the chance to dine on vibrant Indonesian cuisine prepared with nutritional consideration of skilled COMO chefs.

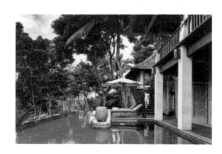

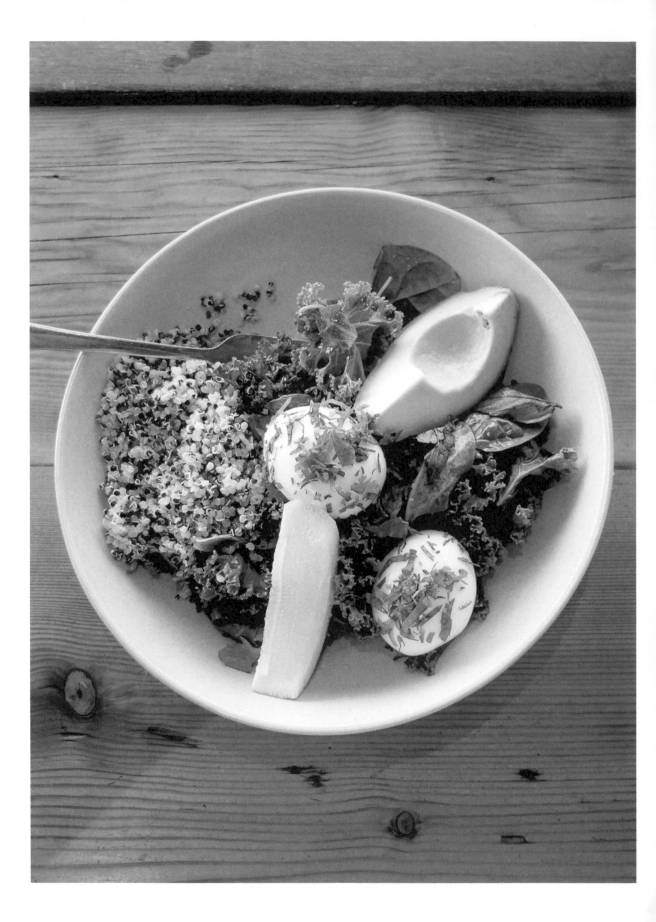

PORCH AND PARLOUR
GREEN BREAKY BOWL

PREPARATION

Dressing:
1) Whisk together coconut oil, lemon zest and juice, and grated turmeric.
2) Let the turmeric infuse into the oil until it starts to turn orange.

Bowl:
1) Wash the kale, Swiss chard, and baby spinach and set aside for cooking.
2) Bring water to boil in a small pot and add eggs for 5 minutes and 30 seconds. Once this time is up, place eggs directly into cool water. Peel and set aside.
3) Bring a nonstick pan to high heat and add washed greens. Continue to stir while adding dressing (the dressing will help the vegetables steam). Don't leave the greens cooking for too long to make sure the leaves stay vibrant and colorful.
4) Place ingredients into bowls. Use wilted greens as a nest for soft boiled eggs, quinoa, avocado quarters, and lemon wedge.
5) Garnish eggs with chopped fresh herbs, salt, and pepper. Drizzle remaining dressing on each dish.

INGREDIENTS

(Serves 4)

Dressing:
- » *Juice and zest of 1 lemon*
- » *1 cup / 220 ml coconut oil*
- » *2 tsp fresh turmeric (grated)*
- » *Salt and pepper to taste*

Bowl:
- » *1 medium bunch of kale*
- » *1 medium bunch of Swiss chard*
- » *3 ⅓ cups / 100 g baby spinach*
- » *1 small bunch of mint*
- » *1 small bunch of parsley*
- » *1 small bunch of cilantro*
- » *2 cups / 370 g cooked white quinoa*
- » *8 eggs*
- » *1 avocado (quartered)*
- » *1 lemon (quartered)*

PORCH AND PARLOUR

Porch and Parlour is a health and locally focused institution. It is filled with hipsters, it-girls, yogis, skaters, and starlets, all enjoying simple, seasonal dishes in a relaxed atmosphere that magically overlooks iconic Bondi Beach.

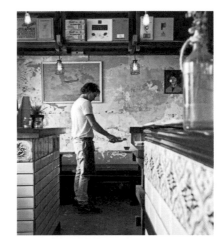

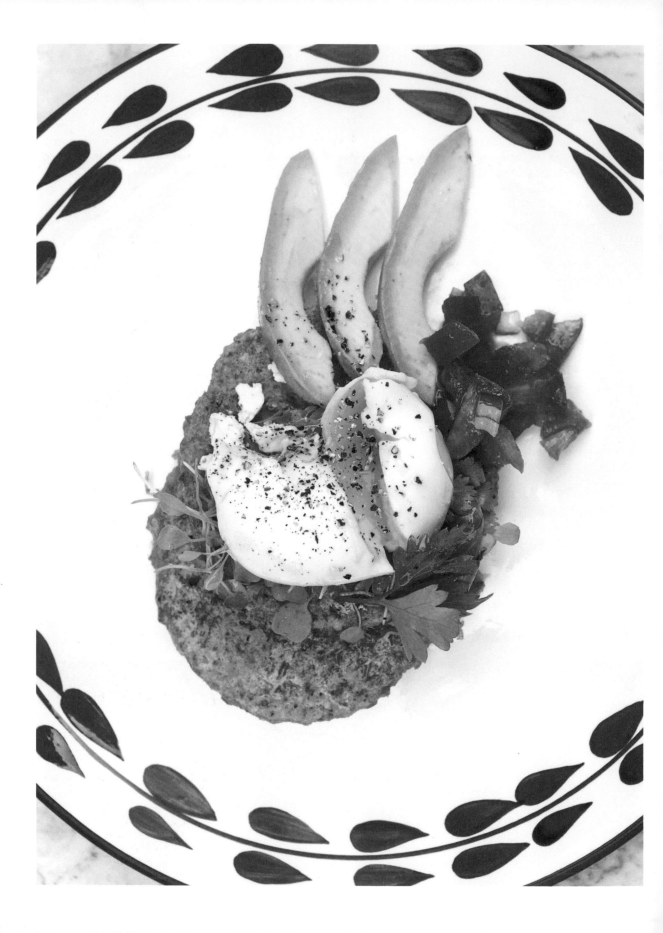

PORCH AND PARLOUR
GREEN PEA PANCAKE

PREPARATION

1) Blanch peas for 10 seconds in boiling water, strain and cool.

2) In a food processor, add blanched peas, red onion, cornstarch, and 2 raw eggs. Pulse the food processor until half the peas are blended. Season as necessary.

3) In a hot nonstick pan, add coconut oil and fry about ¼ of pea mix until golden brown. Flip over and repeat on the other side.

4) Place cooked pea pancake on a plate and garnish with fresh herbs and feta, avocado, and a poached or soft boiled egg. Drizzle with coconut oil.

Note: A nice tomato relish or hot sauce is the perfect accompaniment to this dish.

INGREDIENTS

(For 4 pancakes)

» *3 ⅓ cups / 500 g fresh or frozen green peas*
» *½ red onion (diced)*
» *1 cup / 140 g gluten-free cornstarch*
» *2 eggs*
» *Salt and pepper to taste*

Garnish:
» *1 small bunch of mint*
» *1 small bunch of flat-leaf parsley*
» *1 small bunch of cilantro*
» *¼ cup / 50 g Danish feta*
» *1 avocado (sliced)*
» *4 poached or soft boiled eggs*
» *1 tbsp coconut oil*

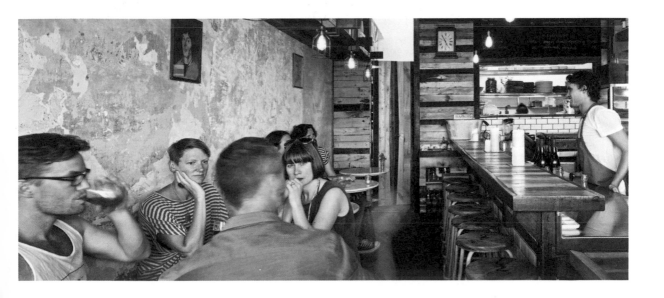

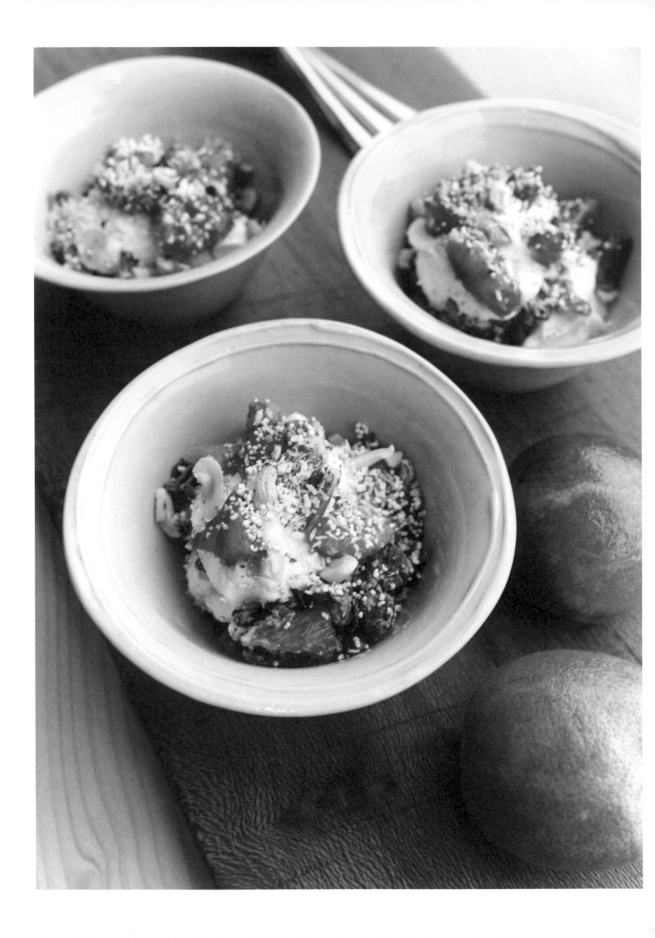

THE STORE KITCHEN
SPROUTED QUINOA & BUCKWHEAT GRANOLA

PREPARATION

1) To sprout the buckwheat and quinoa, wash both well and soak overnight in cold water. After 12 hours, drain the water and leave the grains in separate containers with breathable tops (we use jars with cheesecloth secured over the rim).

2) Wash the grains and drain the water every 12 hours until you see the sprouts growing.

3) To make coconut kefir, use kefir milk grains and culture standard coconut milk or yogurt with these for 24 hours. Then strain the grains from the mix and leave the coconut kefir in the fridge for 12 hours to firm up.

4) The cultured coconut will now be teeming with probiotics and an added sourness which works well against the granola. If it is not possible to make your own kefir, a decent coconut yogurt or the flesh from organic coconut milk would also work, there are some good brands found in health food shops for both of these.

5) Toast the cardamom and cinnamon sticks in a pan until you can smell their aromas.

6) Remove from the pan, grind in a spice grinder or pestle and mortar. Add the ground spices to the mixed quinoa and buckwheat first, then add the uncooked nuts, coconut oil, maple syrup, and salt. You can taste and adjust the sweetness and seasoning at this stage.

7) Preheat the oven to 300°F / 150°C. Place the mix on a lined baking sheet and into the oven. Cook it slow.

8) When the top of the mixture is golden, take it out the oven, give it a mix, and then place it back in the oven. Repeat this until you have the crunch you like. In an airtight container, the granola will keep for 2 weeks.

9) To serve, add layers of the granola, coconut kefir, and blood orange segments to a bowl. Top with blood orange, a final dollop of coconut, a sprinkle of the toasted nuts, and popped amaranth.

INGREDIENTS

(Makes 1 large batch)

» *3 cups / 500 g buckwheat*
» *3 cups / 500 g quinoa*
» *Kefir milk grains (optional)*
» *2 cups / 500 ml coconut milk, coconut yogurt, or flesh from coconut milk*
» *1 cup / 200 ml coconut oil (melted)*
» *⅔ cup / 200 ml maple syrup*
» *6 cardamom pods*
» *3 cinnamon sticks*
» *¾ cup / 100 g almonds*
» *About ⅔ cup / 100 g brazil nuts, cashews, peanuts, or hazelnuts*
» *Large pinch of Himalayan pink salt or coarse sea salt*

Garnish:
» *⅜ cup / 50 g walnuts (chopped and toasted)*
» *¼ cup / 50 g amaranth*
» *1 blood orange (peeled and segmented)*

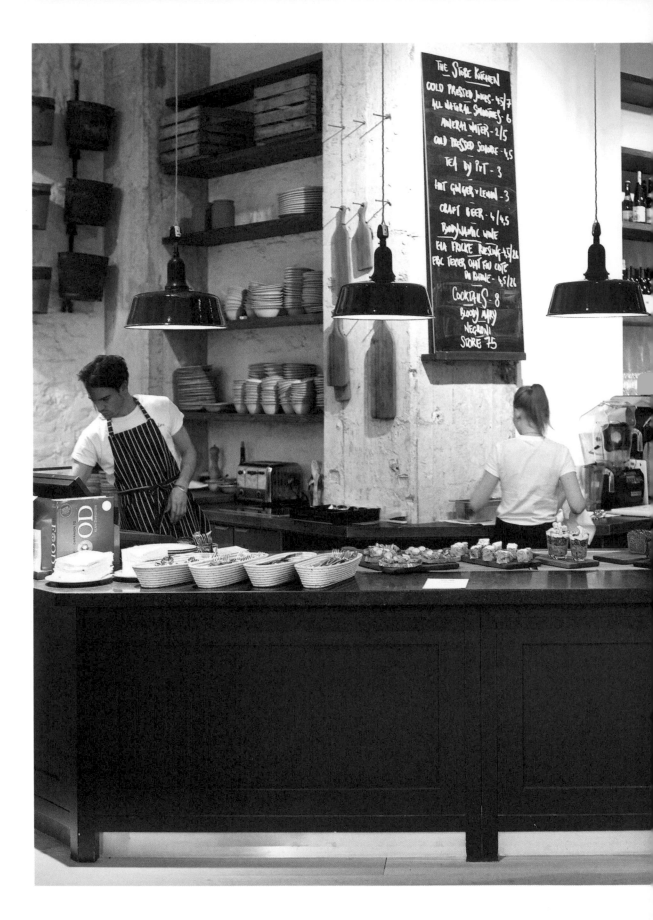

THE STORE KITCHEN

The Store, by creative director Alex Eagle, is a new concept that combines design, furniture, fashion, books, music, art, and food in Berlin. Set inside the space lies The Store Kitchen, a clean organic cafe by day that transforms into a cocktail and wine bar in the evening. In March 2015, Johnnie Collins and Tommy Tannock opened The Store Kitchen with a focus on using quality artisanal products to create fresh and simple, yet delicious, food.

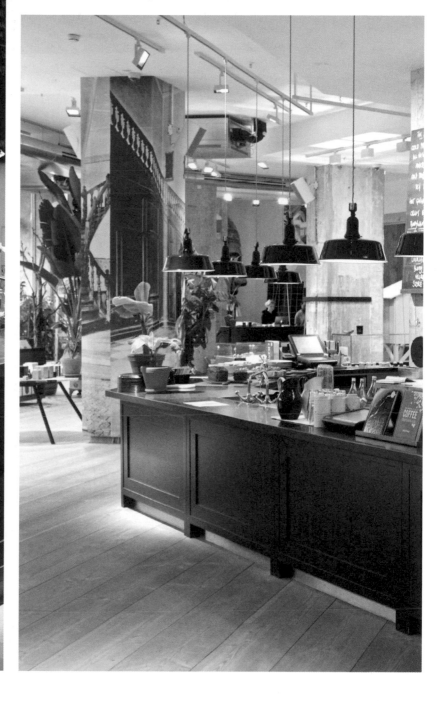

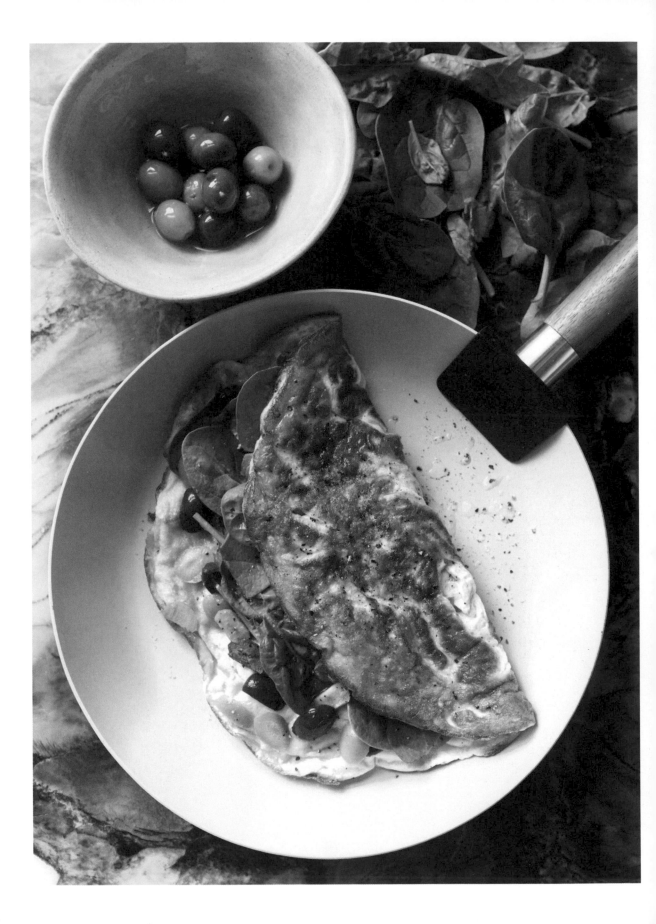

SAMANTHA BRETT
OMELET WITH RICOTTA, OLIVES, & SPINACH

PREPARATION

1) Heat a small round oven-proof omelet pan on the stove on high and preheat oven to 350°F / 180°C.
2) Whisk three eggs together, adding the skim or almond milk bit by bit.
3) When egg mixture is frothy, pour it into a small round omelet pan (you can use olive or coconut oil to line the pan).
4) Wait until bubbles start to form then add small spoons of ricotta, dotting it around the mixture in a circle.
5) Place pan into the oven, leaving the handle out and the oven door open.
6) Wait a few minutes until omelet browns and cheese melts.
7) Remove from the oven and dot olives on top of the ricotta.
8) Pull omelet out of the pan slowly, folding it to one side onto a plate.
9) Top off with a handful of spinach. Add salt and pepper to taste and a drizzle of olive oil.

INGREDIENTS

» 3 eggs
» 2 tbsp skim ricotta
» 2 tbsp skim milk or almond milk
» 1 handful of baby spinach
» 1 handful of pitted olives
» Salt, pepper, and olive oil to taste

SAMANTHA BRETT

Samantha Brett is a news reporter as well as an international best-selling author and journalist living in Sydney. She is the author of six books on dating and relationships and believes healthy living, cooking, and sharing good food are the best ways to keep the spark alive in any relationship.

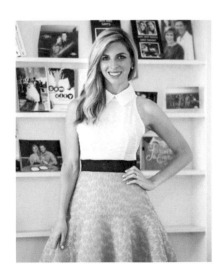

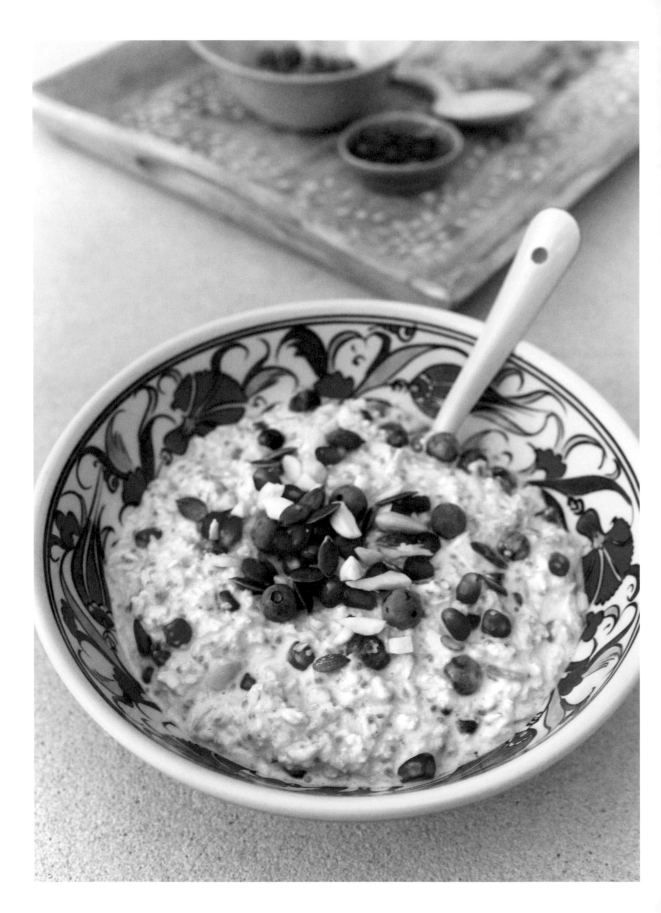

TALI SHINE
SUMMER BIRCHER MUESLI

PREPARATION

1) Add oats, apple juice, coconut milk, and chia seeds to a bowl and gently stir to combine.

2) Place the bowl in refrigerator and soak overnight.

3) Place a small amount of the coconut, almonds, pumpkin seeds, pomegranate, and blueberries aside for garnish.

4) In the morning, mix in the grated apples, coconut yogurt, maple syrup, shredded coconut, almonds, pumpkin seeds, blueberries, pomegranate seeds, and cinnamon.

5) Refrigerate for an hour.

6) Garnish with the seeds, nuts, fruits, and coconut that were put to the side.

INGREDIENTS

» 2 cups / 180 g gluten-free oats
» 2 tbsp white chia seeds
» 2 cups / 480 ml fresh apple juice
» 3 tbsp coconut milk
» 2 tbsp sliced almonds
» 2 tbsp shredded coconut
» 2 tbsp pumpkin seeds
» 1 ½ cups / 350 g coconut yogurt
» 1 tbsp maple syrup
» 2 Granny Smith apples (grated)
» 1 cup / 150 g fresh pomegranate seeds
» 1 cup / 130 g fresh blueberries
» Cinnamon to taste

TALI SAYS:

"Summer bircher muesli is my family's favorite morning dish. Made in a large batch or individual shot glasses for entertaining, it is delicious and looks beautiful. Kids and adults will all come back for seconds!"

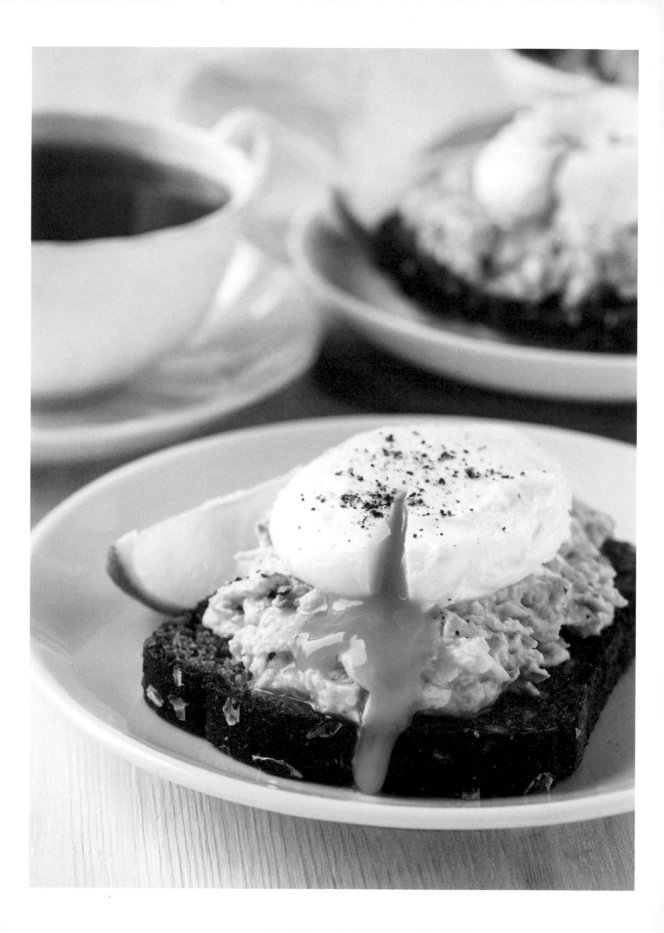

STEPH ADAMS
POACHED EGGS, SMASHED AVO

PREPARATION

1) Poach the eggs for about 3 minutes.

2) Toast two pieces of gluten-free bread.

3) Use a fork to smash avocado and then place on to the toast. Add the olive oil and chopped basil.

4) Place the poached eggs on top of the avocado and halve so that the yolks run across the avocado and toast.

5) Top with chopped chives and serve.

Note: A nice tomato relish or chopped cherry tomatoes are the perfect accompaniment to this dish.

INGREDIENTS

» *2 eggs*
» *2 pieces of gluten-free toast*
» *1 avocado*
» *1 tbsp olive oil*
» *2 tbsp basil (chopped)*
» *2 tbsp chives (chopped)*
» *Pinch of rock salt*
» *8 cherry tomatoes (chopped in halves) (optional)*

STEPH SAYS:

"This dish is such a rich source of protein and tastes so good."

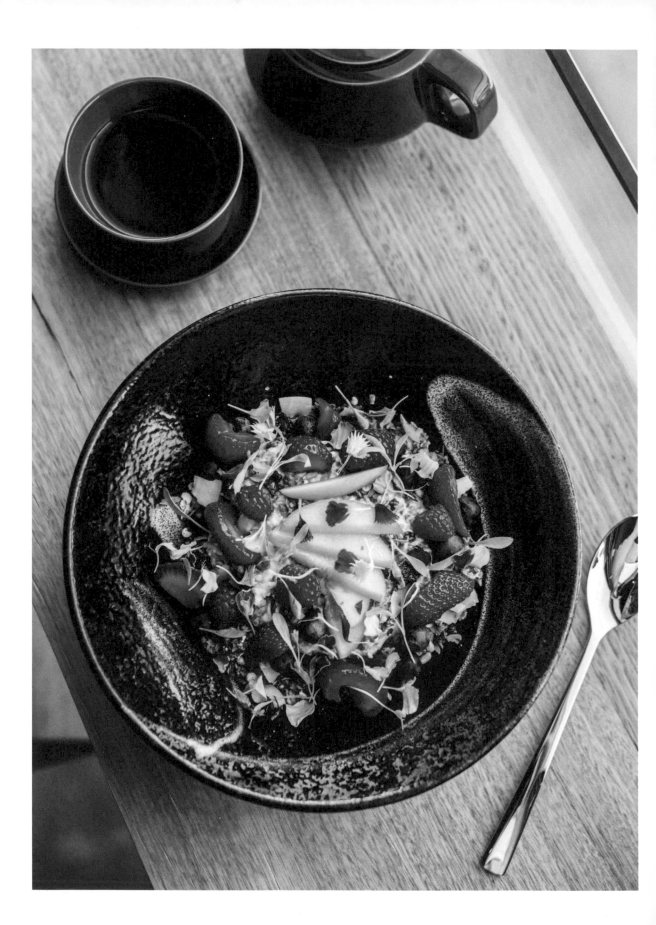

HARRY'S BONDI
COCONUT
CHIA PUDDING

PREPARATION

1) Whisk coconut milk and agave nectar together with chia seeds and allow to bloom in the fridge for two hours.

2) Whisk in coconut yogurt and allow to set overnight.

3) Serve with raw granola, edible flowers, and seasonal fruits.

INGREDIENTS

» 1 ¾ cups / 400 ml coconut milk
» 1 ⅓ tbsp agave or coconut nectar
» ⅓ cup / 60 g white chia seeds
» 2 cups and 1 tbsp / 500 g coconut yogurt
» Raw granola, edible flowers, seasonal fruits for garnish

HARRY'S BONDI

Offering relaxed hospitality and a buzzing vibe with a backdrop of the iconic Bondi Beach, Harry's Bondi is an approachable Sydney hot spot that focuses on clean eating with a modern twist. The seasonally changing menu showcases whole food items that satisfy guests over leisurely breakfasts and long lunches every day of the week.

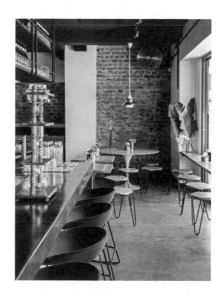

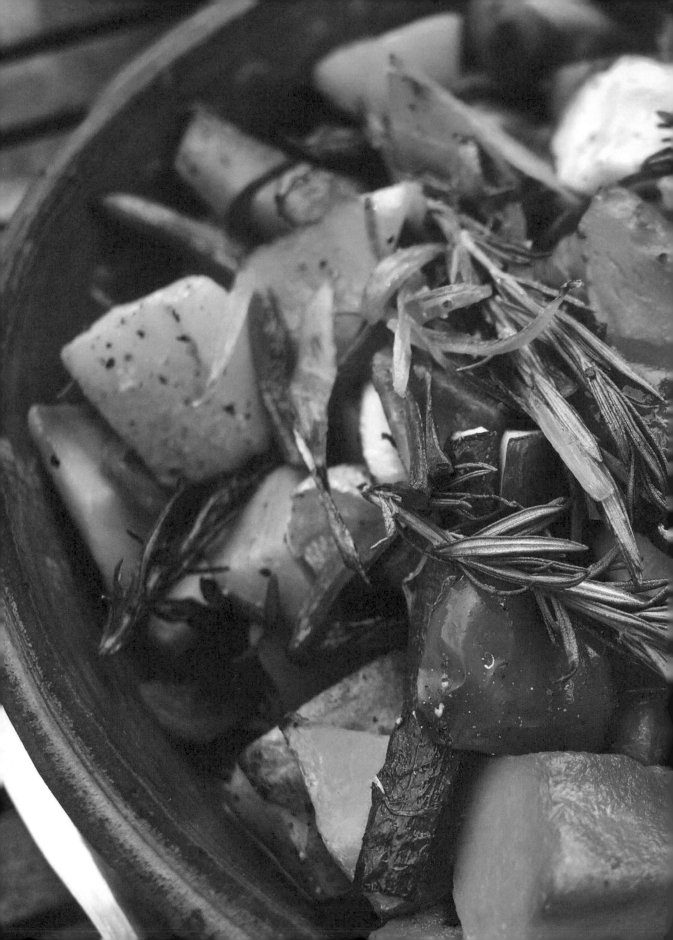

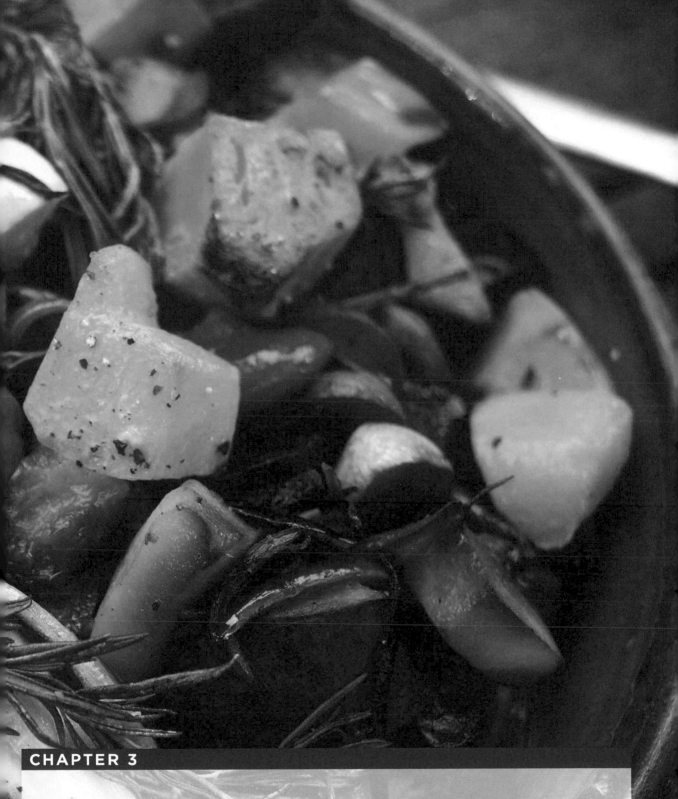

CHAPTER 3

SALADS & MAINS

DIG IN!

Whether dining alone or cooking for friends and family, you'll love these delicious dishes that feed the soul and satisfy the stomach. These recipes work year round and feature salads that make appetizing starter dishes or fantastic standalone meals.

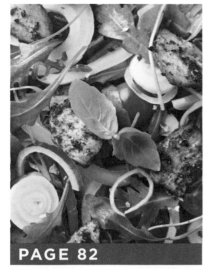

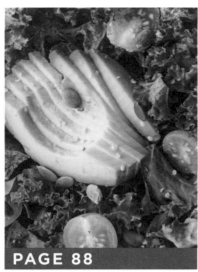

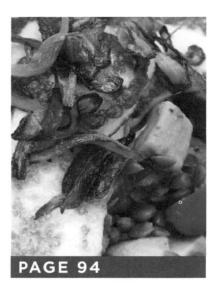

PAGE 82

PAGE 88

PAGE 94

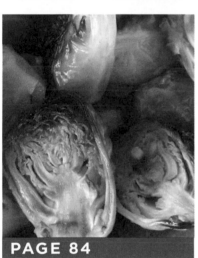

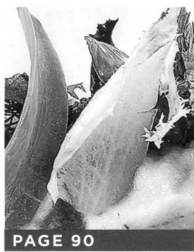

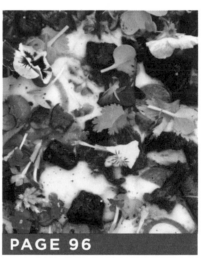

PAGE 84

PAGE 90

PAGE 96

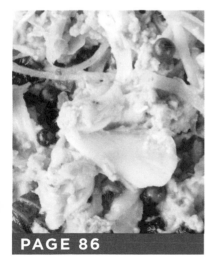

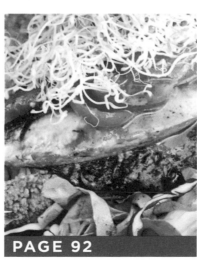

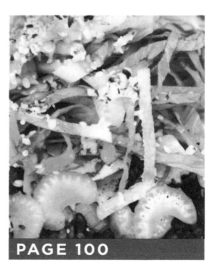

PAGE 86

PAGE 92

PAGE 100

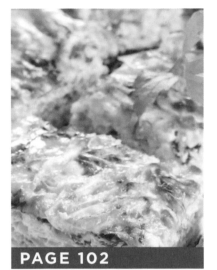

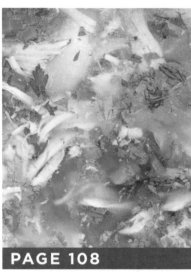

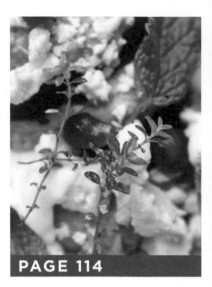

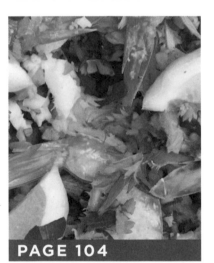

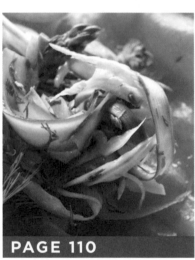

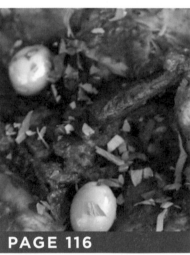

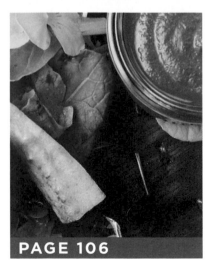

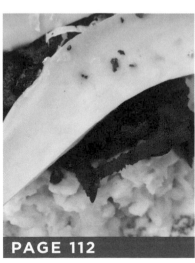

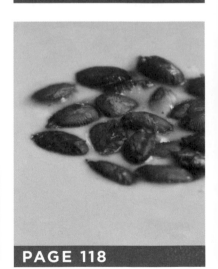

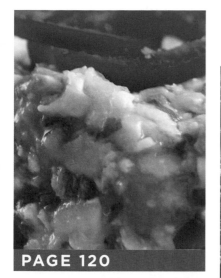

PAGE 120

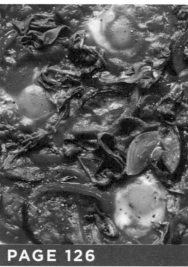

PAGE 126

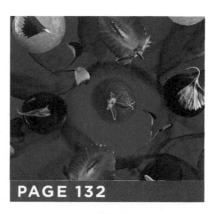

PAGE 132

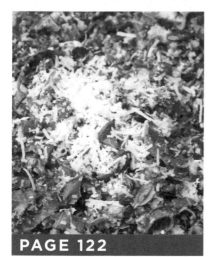

PAGE 122

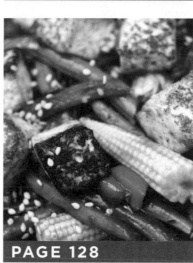

PAGE 128

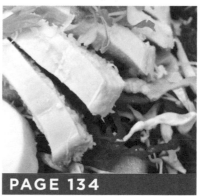

PAGE 134

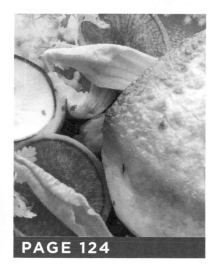

PAGE 124

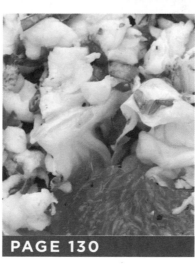

PAGE 130

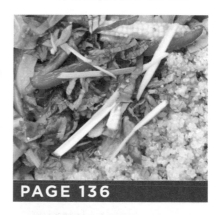

PAGE 136

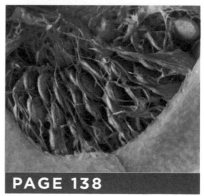

PAGE 138

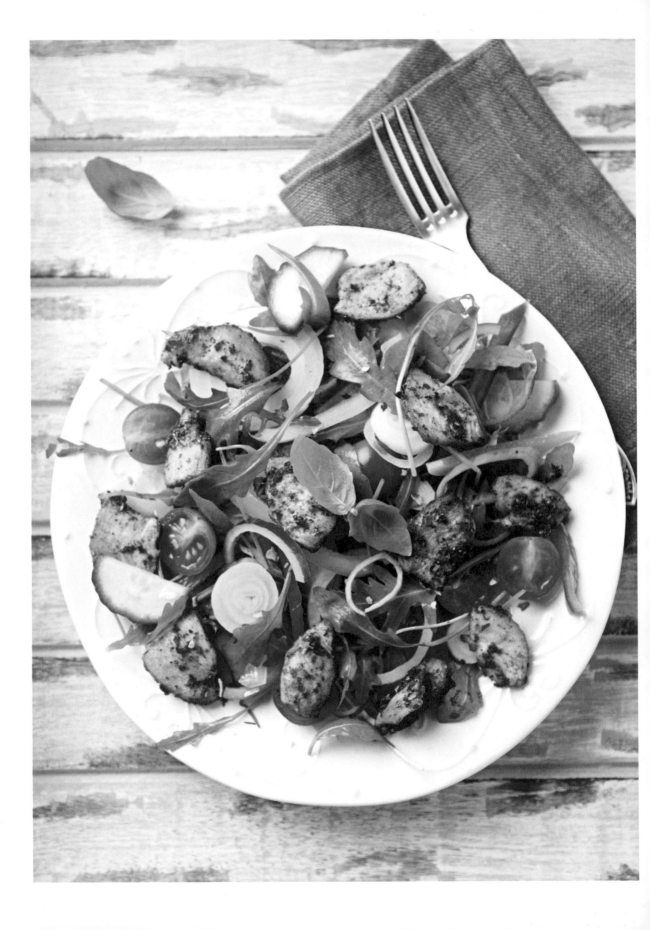

LISA CLAYTON
LEMON, COCONUT, & ROSEMARY CHICKEN

PREPARATION

1) Coat chicken breast in coconut flour, then egg.

2) Cover with desiccated coconut, fresh rosemary, and lemon zest (ratio 3:2:1).

3) Shallow fry in ghee or coconut oil.

4) Serve with spinach (or arugula), basil, onion, tomato, bell pepper, and cucumber.

5) Drizzle with lemon juice and olive oil.

6) Salt and pepper to taste.

INGREDIENTS

» 3–4 chicken breasts
» 1 egg
» Coconut flour
» ½ cup / 45 g desiccated coconut
» ½ cup / 15 g rosemary (chopped)
» 4 tbsp lemon zest
» Coconut oil or ghee
» 3 cups / 90 g spinach
» ¼ cup / 10 g basil leaves
   (or arugula or baby leaf greens)
» ¼ onion (chopped)
» 1 handful of cherry tomatoes (halved)
» ½ red bell pepper (slivered)
» ½ cucumber (sliced)
» ¼ cup / 60 ml lemon juice
» 2 tbsp of olive oil
» Pinch of salt
» Pinch of pepper

LISA CLAYTON

Lisa Clayton co-founded Singapore's largest outdoor fitness community, UFIT Bootcamps and today serves as the company's director in addition to managing SHEFIT, a hugely popular activewear brand for women. The ISSA certified personal trainer started her business so that people living in Singapore could enjoy the benefits of outdoor training in a fun, group environment. Lisa has done lifestyle TV segments for Healthy Me TV, AusBiz Asia, Channel News Asia, and has been featured by magazines including *Women's Health* Australia, *Expat Living*, *Liv*, and *Wellbeing* Australia.

www.ufitbootcamps.com.sg

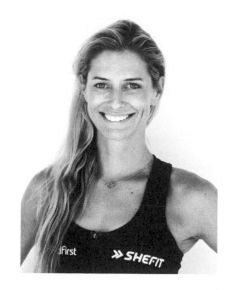

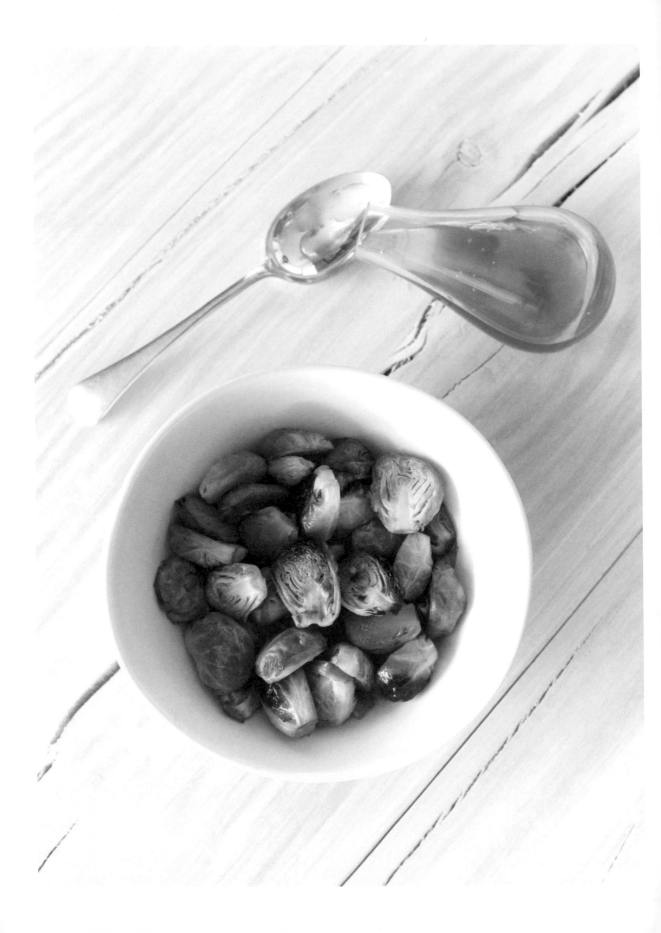

CAFÉ GRATITUDE
ROASTED BRUSSELS SPROUTS IN A MAPLE MISO GLAZE

PREPARATION

1) In a blender, combine the olive oil, maple syrup, red miso, tamari, and apple cider vinegar to make the glaze.

2) Dress the Brussels sprouts liberally with the glaze. Make sure the Brussels are well-coated and lay out on a baking tray. Drizzle ¼ cup / 60 ml of water over the Brussels sprouts to add some vapor while cooking.

3) Bake at 325°F / 160°C for 20 minutes or until well-cooked.

4) Approximately 10 minutes into the cooking time, turn the vegetables to ensure even cooking.

INGREDIENTS

» 3 lbs / 1.4 kg Brussels sprouts (cleaned and cut in half)
» 1 cup / 220 ml olive oil
» ⅓ cup / 110 ml maple syrup
» ½ cup / 140 g red miso
» 1 tbsp tamari soy sauce
» ½ cup / 120 ml apple cider vinegar

CAFÉ GRATITUDE

Celebrity favorite Café Gratitude is a buzzing group of 100% organic, gourmet vegan restaurants in Southern California. The Café Gratitude ethos is about supporting local farmers, sustainable agriculture, and environmentally friendly products, and creating mouth-watering dishes prepared with love.

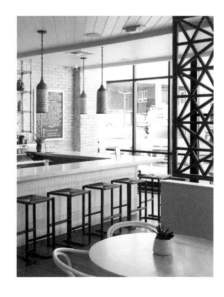

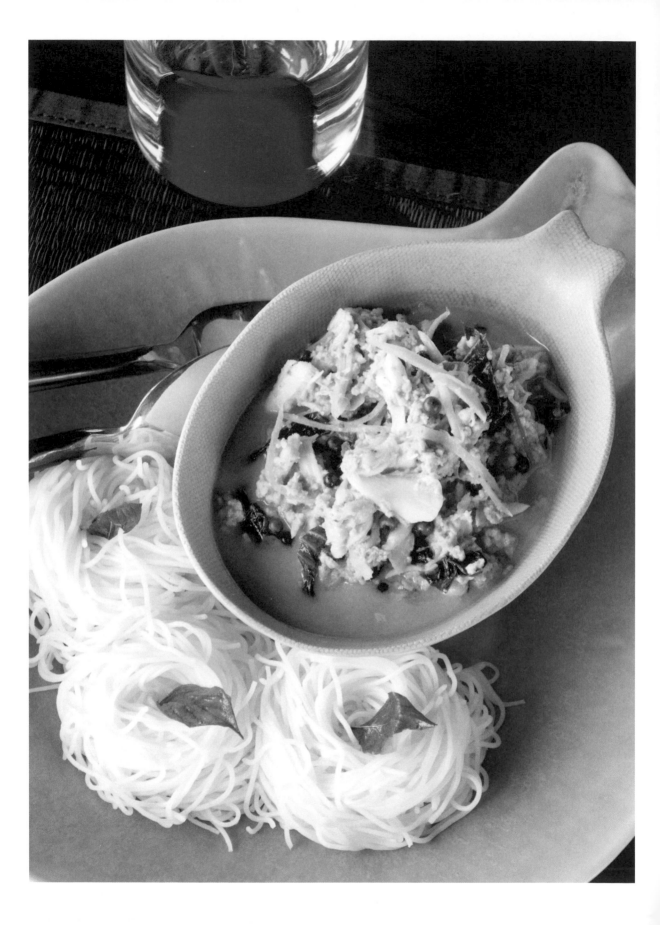

POINT YAMU BY COMO
BLUE CRAB CURRY

PREPARATION

1) To make the red curry paste, combine all ingredients and pound into a paste. Set aside.

2) Heat coconut milk in a pot on the stove until thick. Add red curry paste and stir until it becomes increasingly aromatic.

3) Add ginger, turmeric, and young peppercorn seasoning, then add fish sauce and crab meat.

4) Add betel leaf and stir together.

5) Put curry into a bowl and garnish with young peppercorns.

6) Served with rice noodle and fried sweet basil.

POINT YAMU BY COMO

With sweeping views of the jewel-colored Andaman Sea, Point Yamu by COMO is one of the best resorts in Thailand to retreat—and eat. The resort offers an array of restaurants to choose from, including COMO Shambhala Cuisine that focuses on health.

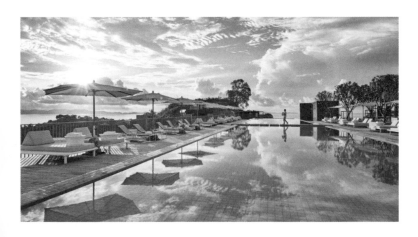

INGREDIENTS

» ½ cup / 100 g crab meat
» ¾ cup and 1 tbsp / 200 ml fresh coconut milk
» ½ cup / 30 g young ginger (peeled, julienned)
» ⅜ cup / 20 g fresh turmeric (peeled, julienned)
» 2 tbsp young peppercorn (seeds only)
» 0.7 oz / 20 g Asian betel leaf (sliced)
» 1 tsp red chili paste (see below)
» 1 tsp fish sauce
» 2 oz / 50 g dried small rice noodle, soak in water and blanch until soft
» ⅛ cup / 2 g sweet basil (fried)

Red Curry Paste:
» ⅔ tsp dried red chili, soak in water 1 h
» 0.1 oz / 3 g dried red chili finger, soak in water 1 h
» 1 small piece galangal (peeled, sliced)
» 0.4 oz / 10 g lemongrass (sliced)
» 1 tsp kaffir lime fruit zest
» ½ tbsp cilantro root
» ½ tbsp Thai shallot (peeled)
» 1 clove Thai garlic
» 3 tsp fresh turmeric (peeled, sliced)
» ⅛ cup / 10 g cilantro seed (roasted)
» ⅛ cup / 12 g cumin seed (roasted)
» ⅛ cup / 13 g black pepper seed
» 1 tsp shrimp paste
» ½ tsp salt

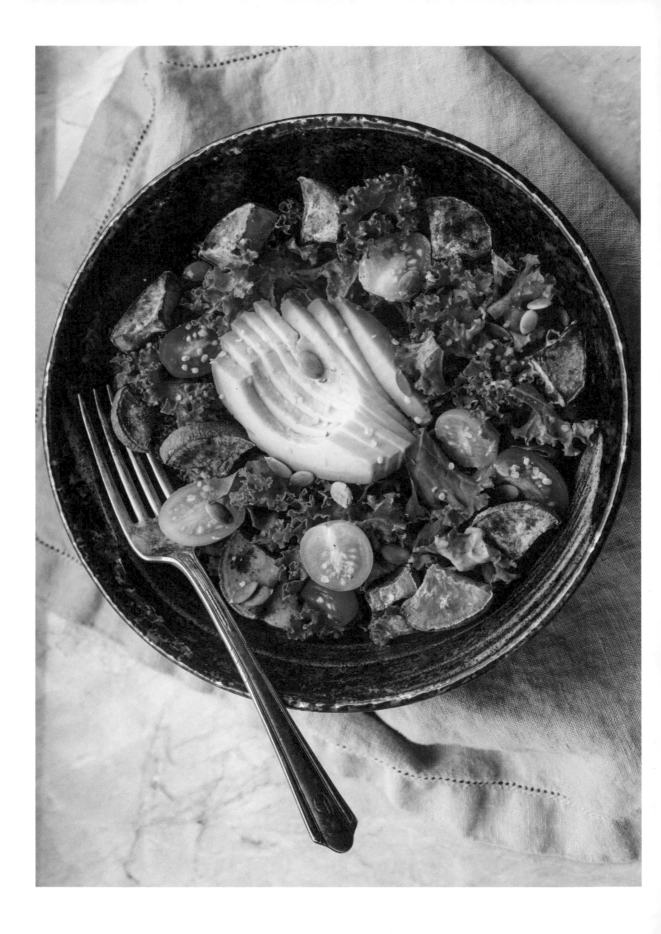

ASHLEA TALBOT
SUPERFOOD SALAD

PREPARATION

1) Remove tough stems from the kale leaves and wash well.

2) Shred finely and place into a bowl.

3) Combine the salt, pepper, lemon juice, dulse flakes, turmeric, olive oil, and vinegar into a small bowl or cup.

4) Whisk the dressing ingredients well, then pour over the shredded kale leaves.

5) Combine the dressing with the kale and massage the leaves gently for a minute, or until the leaves begin to soften.

6) Add the rest of the ingredients for the salad, toss through gently and enjoy.

INGREDIENTS

Kale Salad:
» *1 bunch of kale*
» *½ head broccoli (steamed)*
» *½ cup / 90 g cooked quinoa*
» *10 cubes pumpkin (roasted)*
» *½ avocado (sliced)*
» *10 green beans (steamed)*
» *2 tbsp canned chickpeas*
» *Cucumber (steamed)*
» *Carrot (grated)*
» *1 tsp pepitas*
» *1 tsp goji berries*
» *Sprinkle of edible flowers (optional)*
» *4 cherry tomatoes (cut) (optional)*

Dressing:
» *5 tsp extra-virgin olive oil*
» *2 tsp champagne vinegar*
» *1 dash lemon juice*
» *Pinch of Himalayan pink salt*
» *Pinch of pepper*
» *Pinch of turmeric*
» *Pinch of dulse flakes*

ASHLEA TALBOT

Ashlea Talbot is an internationally-accredited yoga teacher with more than 350 hours of teacher training in Ashtanga Vinyasa yoga, power yoga, as well as both pre and post natal yoga. Before Ashlea began her yoga career she worked around the world as a model, TV presenter, and was crowned Miss Universe Australia in 2003. Ashlea has hosted television shows and starred in commercials for brands such as Toyota, Tourism Australia, and more.

www.ashleatalbot.com

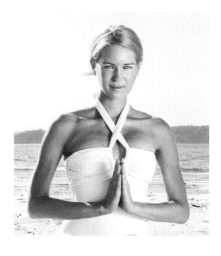

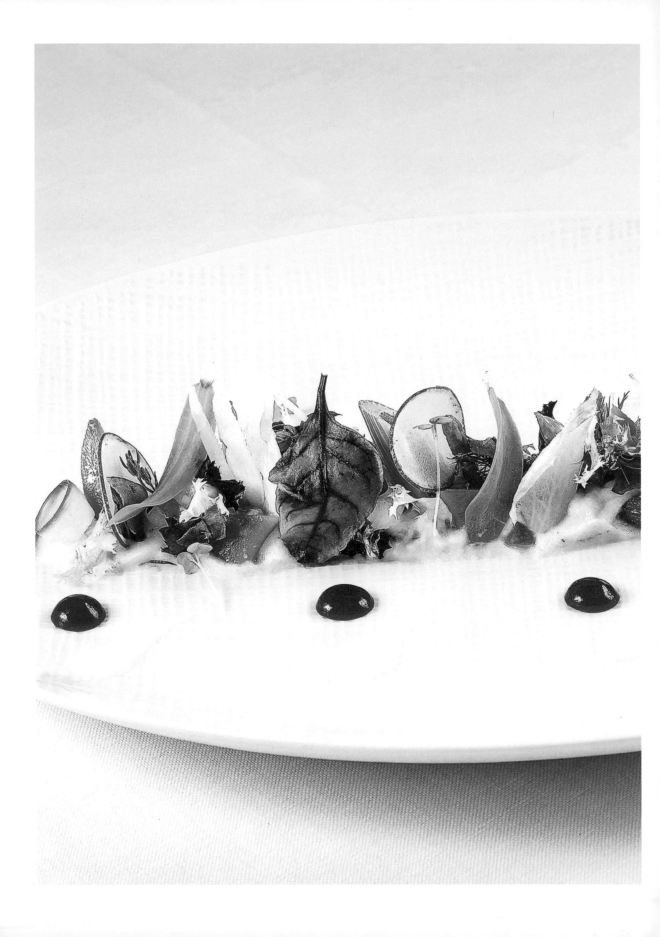

CAPRI PALACE HOTEL & SPA
COTTO E CRUDO DI VERDURE

PREPARATION

1) Cut the eggplants in half and place a peeled garlic clove in the center.
2) Garnish with thyme and olive oil and wrap with aluminum foil.
3) Oven bake at 350°F / 180°C for 1 hour.
4) Cut the red onion in brunoise shape (small cubes) and blanch in hot water.
5) Wash and mince the parsley, then squeeze with a cloth.
6) Cut the tomato fillet into brunoise.
7) Empty the eggplants by taking the pulp away and drain it in a strainer.
8) Chop the eggplant skin thinly. Chop the eggplant pulp as well.
9) Sear the anchovies with a bit of olive oil in a frying pan.
10) Add the eggplant skin and pulp to the anchovies.
11) Take away from heat and finish with capers, tomato cubes, parsley, onion, olive oil, Barolo vinegar, and raw and cooked vegetables.
12) Season to taste.

INGREDIENTS

Eggplant "Caviar":
- » *4 ½ lbs / 2 kg eggplants*
- » *2 garlic cloves for each eggplant*
- » *4 sprigs lemon thyme*
- » *1 red onion*
- » *½ bunch of parsley*
- » *8 tomato fillets*
- » *2 salted anchovies*
- » *½ tbsp capers*
- » *1 ½ tbsp Barolo red wine vinegar*
- » *Salt, pepper, extra-virgin olive oil to taste*
- » *Raw vegetables, sliced thinly (carrots, fennel, celery, asparagus, radish)*
- » *Cooked vegetables (carrots, zucchini, asparagus, broad beans, green peas)*

Garnish:
- » *Flowers for decoration (violet)*
- » *Deep-fried celeriac slice*
- » *Balsamic vinegar dressing*

CAPRI PALACE HOTEL & SPA

The Capri Palace Hotel & Spa is a luxury hotel of refined elegance that recalls an ancient Neapolitan palace of the 1700s. Everything served is made with exclusively 100% organic and local ingredients. The resort is just steps away from the small and charming center of Anacapri, an authentic village on the charming island of Capri.

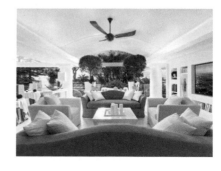

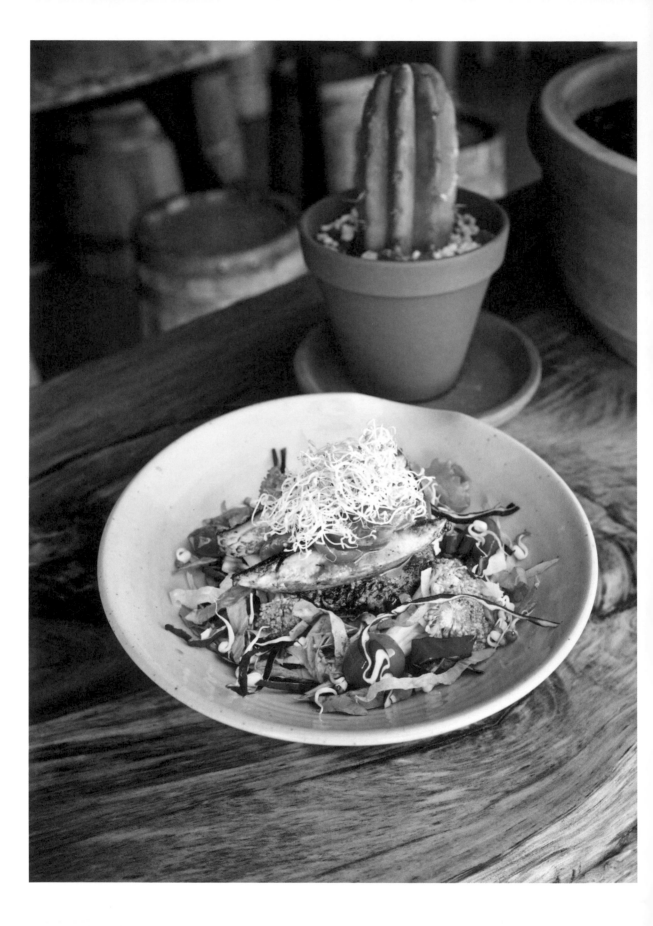

SEXY FOOD
SEXY BUN-LESS BURGER

PREPARATION

Black Bean and Mushroom Veg Patty:

1) Blend and mash the black beans. Roughly blitz the raw mushroom, then the leeks and carrots together, and add the rest of the ingredients. Season to taste and carefully shape into sexy patties.

2) Pan fry patties in coconut oil, macadamia oil or virgin olive oil over medium heat until crispy and light brown on both sides.

Raw Tomato Relish:

1) For the relish, mix all ingredients together.

To Serve:

1) Serve everything on a bed of mixed leafy greens, live cultured sauerkraut or kimchi, steamed broccoli and cauliflower, or cultured kefir cheese with relish on the side.

2) Garnish with fresh alfalfa sprouts.

INGREDIENTS

Black Bean and Mushroom Veg Patty:
- » ½ cup / 40 g black beans (soaked overnight, then boiled for 30 mins)
- » 1 cup / 100 g mushrooms
- » 1 cup / 50 g leeks and carrots (diced)
- » ¾ cup / 70 g gluten-free oats
- » 2 tbsp nutritional yeast
- » ½ tbsp tamari soy sauce
- » ½ tsp Himalayan pink salt
- » ½ tsp ground cumin
- » ⅛–¼ cup / 5–10 g fresh cilantro
- » ⅛–¼ cup / 5–10 g fresh parsley
- » 1 ¾ tbsp fresh rosemary
- » ¼ tsp ground pepper
- » 1 egg

Raw Tomato Relish:
- » ½ cup / 50 g sun-dried tomatoes (soaked overnight)
- » ⅛ cup / 25 g dates (soaked overnight)
- » ¼ cup / 15 g parsley
- » 2 tbsp rosemary
- » ½ cup / 100 ml virgin olive oil
- » 5 tsp apple cider vinegar
- » 2 tsp tamari soy sauce
- » Pinch of chili powder
- » ½ tsp Himalayan pink salt

To Serve:
- » Leafy greens
- » Live cultured sauerkraut or kimchi
- » Broccoli and cauliflower (steamed)
- » Cultured kefir cheese (optional)
- » Alfalfa sprouts

SEXY FOOD

Cape Town's sexiest spot for organic, healthy fare, Sexy Food serves wholesome, nutritionally-packed goodness worthy of your Instagram feed. Owner James Kuiper's Bree Street eatery is famed for its gluten-free veggie burger, abundance bowls, and fresh pressed juices. Guests can even cut their own micro greens—it doesn't get any fresher!

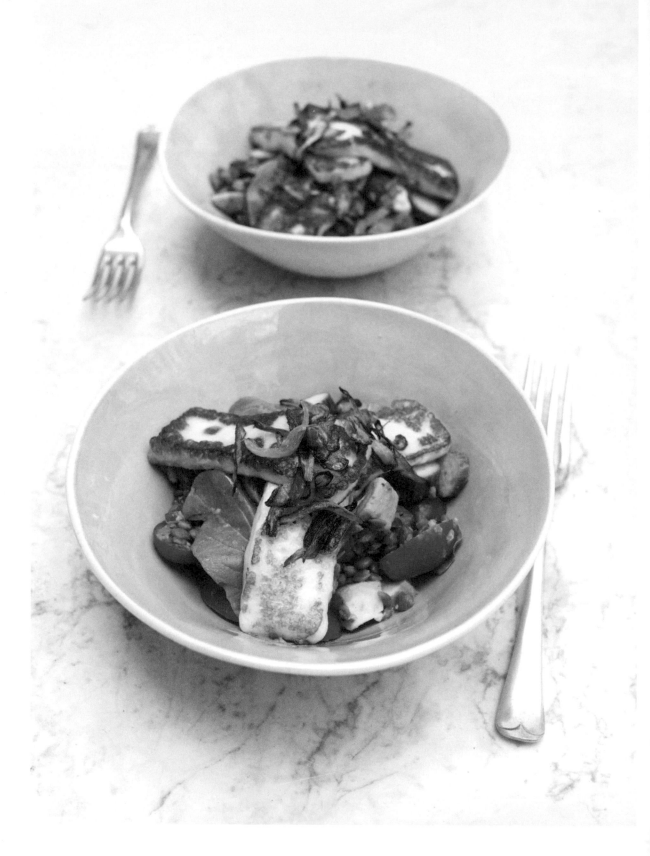

TALI SHINE
HALLOUMI & BROWN LENTIL SALAD

PREPARATION

1) Slice onion and fry until brown. Combine with lentils.

2) Mix the lentils, onion, tomatoes, avocado, cucumber, and rocket in a bowl and season with olive oil, salt, and pepper.

3) Arrange onto plates.

4) Heat a pan with coconut oil, squeeze lemon onto the halloumi slices and fry until lightly brown, about 1–2 minutes on each side.

5) Pat dry with a paper towel and squeeze lemon over.

6) Arrange halloumi slices onto plated salads.

INGREDIENTS

(Serves 2)

» 2 ¼ cups / 400 g brown lentils (soaked and cooked)
» ¼ onion
» 1 small package cherry tomatoes (halved)
» 2 Lebanese cucumbers (sliced)
» 1 avocado (diced)
» 1 bunch of baby arugula (rocket) leaves
» Olive oil
» Coconut oil
» 1 package sheep's milk halloumi (sliced)
» Juice of 1 lemon

TALI SAYS:

"This is the perfect hearty salad, and what I make when I need that extra protein. I always add a little apple cider vinegar to the lentils, as this helps to make the digestion easier."

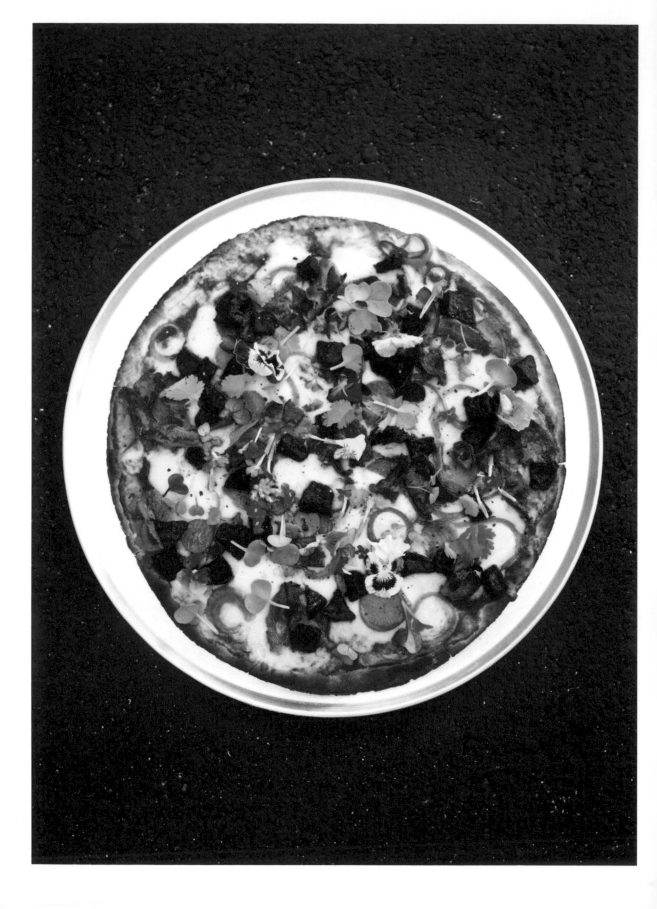

ARCADE CAFÉ
SOHO PIZZA

Pickled Red Onion and Radish Dressing:

1) Combine all wet ingredients, salt, and honey and mix well.

2) Slice red onion and radishes. Add into a bowl with vinegar mix and let pickle for a day or longer.

Note: Try adding dried chili flakes or various herbs to play with the pickle flavor.

Tomato Base:

1) Using a hand blender or food processor, add all tomato base ingredients together and blend into a smooth puree.

2) Set aside to slather on pizza dough.

Note: To add different depths of flavors to the base sauce, add nutmeg or dried chili flakes.

Roasted Beets:

1) Preheat oven to 480°F / 250°C.

2) Mix all ingredients together thoroughly. Roast in the oven for approximately 20 minutes until beets are cooked, but still have a raw crunch.

Pickled Red Onion and Radish Dressing:
- » *½ red onion*
- » *1–2 radishes*
- » *2 cups and 1 tbsp / 500 ml white wine vinegar*
- » *2 cups and 1 tbsp / 500 ml red wine vinegar*
- » *1 ¼ cups / 250 ml extra-virgin olive oil*
- » *1 cup / 250 ml fresh lemon or lime juice (lime will be a little sweeter)*
- » *3 tbsp salt*
- » *¼ cup / 80 g honey (or agave nectar or maple syrup)*
- » *Dried chili flakes or various herbs (optional)*

Tomato Base:
- » *5.5 lbs / 2.5 kg whole peeled tomatoes*
- » *4 ½ tbsp dried oregano*
- » *1 ½ tbsp Maldon sea salt*
- » *2 cups / 50 g fresh basil leaves*
- » *½ cup and 1 tbsp / 120 ml extra-virgin olive oil*
- » *Nutmeg or dried chili flakes (optional)*

Roasted Beets:
- » *1 ⅔ cups / 250 g raw beets (diced)*
- » *1 tbsp extra-virgin olive oil*
- » *¼ cup / 60 ml balsamic vinegar*
- » *1 tbsp honey (or agave nectar or maple syrup)*
- » *Big pinch of salt*

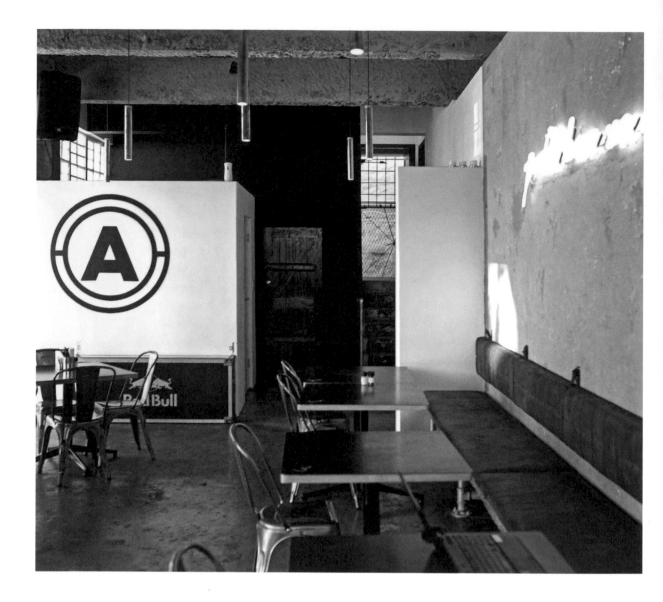

ARCADE CAFÉ

Located on the corner of Bree and Pepper Streets in Cape Town, South Africa, Arcade Café is a bar and restaurant focused on bringing people together for the sake of food, drinks, and socializing. Splurge on cocktails like a Banana Daiquiri and a burger, or keep things light with the hotspot's mixed salads.

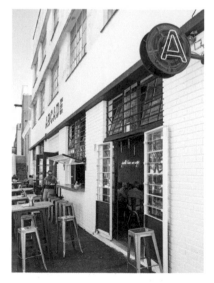

PREPARATION

Roast Garlic Olive Oil:

1) Preheat oven to 390°F / 200°C.

2) Roast garlic in oven until shells turn a light, golden brown color.

3) Remove from the oven and allow to cool. The garlic will sweat inside and cook out all the harsh flavors.

4) Blend extra-virgin olive oil, a pinch of good salt, squeeze of fresh lemon and blend until smooth.

5) Strain ingredients and use to drizzle over finished pizza.

Note: there will be leftover oil. Keep for future barbecue use.

To Serve:

1) Preheat oven to 390°F / 200°C for a gluten-free dough (525°F / 275°C for conventional dough).

2) Assemble pizza dough with tomato sauce, cheese, and beets.

3) Cook pizza in oven for approximately 3–5 minutes.

4) Remove pizza from the oven. Slice pizza and garnish with pickled vegetables, fresh cilantro leaves, and some micro greens to your liking. Finish with a squeeze of lime and drizzle of roasted garlic olive oil.

INGREDIENTS

Roast Garlic Olive Oil:

» *½ cup / 50 g garlic cloves in their shells*
» *2 ½ cups / 500 ml extra-virgin olive oil*
» *Pinch of salt*
» *Juice of 1 lemon*

To Serve:

» *Store-bought gluten-free pizza dough (many options are available online or at your local health food store. We prefer the bases made from tapioca and rice flour as opposed to the cauliflower bases.)*
» *1 big ladle of tomato base about ½ cup / 100 ml*
» *3.5 oz / 100 g mozzarella*
» *4 oz / 120 g mozzarella fior di latte*
» *Roasted beets*
» *Pickled vegetables*
» *Cilantro for garnish and micro greens of your choice*
» *1 lime for garnish*
» *Roast garlic olive oil*
» *Baking stone (preferably a granite slab) to simulate a pizza oven*

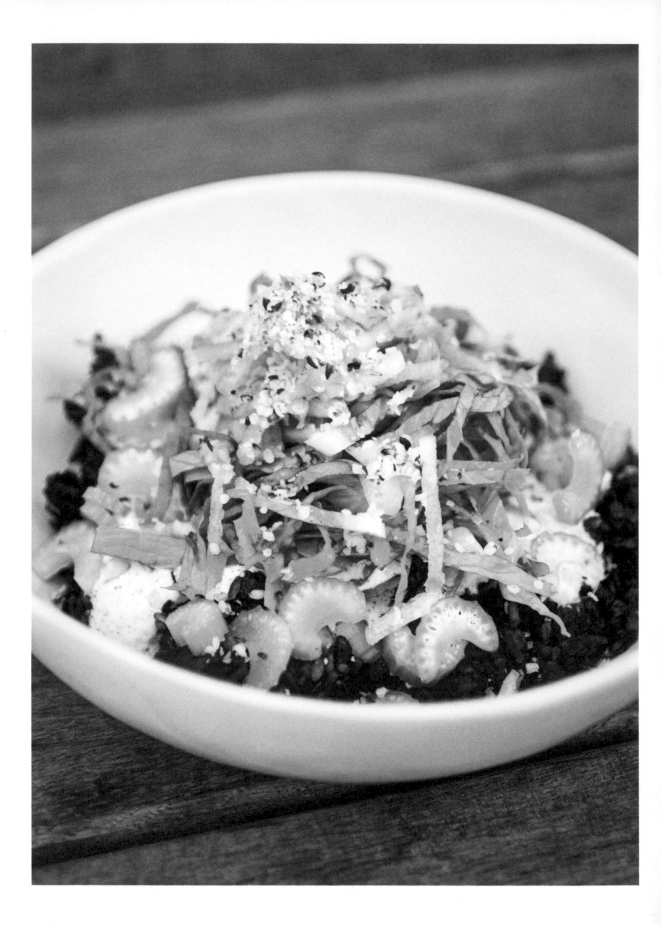

DALUMA
APPLE HEMP CREAM
WITH BELUGA LENTILS

PREPARATION

Beluga Lentils:
1) Rinse lentils under running water.
2) Bring water to a boil, add lentils and lower to medium heat.
3) Let simmer for 15 to 20 minutes, when almost done add salt. Set aside.

Apple Hemp Cream:
1) Rinse apples, remove stems, and cut into cubes.
2) Add all ingredients into a high-speed blender and blend until completely smooth. Add more water (up to ⅞ cup / 200 ml) if you prefer a thinner sauce.

To Serve:
1) Cut celery and romaine hearts into thin slices.
2) Grate apples roughly.
3) Juice lemon and pour over grated apples. Mix lemon zest with hemp seeds.
4) Distribute lentils on pre-warmed plates.
5) Scoop out a hole in the middle of the lentils to pour sauce.
6) Arrange in the following order: apple hemp cream, celery, romaine hearts, grated apples, and hemp seeds.

INGREDIENTS

Beluga Lentils:
» *2 cups / 400 g Beluga lentils*
» *Salt to taste*

Apple Hemp Cream:
» *8.5 oz / 240 g apple*
» *2 ½ cups / 600 g hemp seeds*
» *2 ½ cups / 600 ml filtered water*
» *2 tbsp nutritional yeast*
» *½ cup / 140 ml fresh lemon juice*
» *1 tbsp garlic (grated)*
» *4 tsp salt*

Garnish:
» *2 romaine hearts*
» *2 apples*
» *Juice and zest of 1 lemon*
» *2 stalks celery*
» *1 cup / 240 g hemp seeds*

DALUMA

Daluma is a Berlin health food hotspot located nearby Rosenthaler Platz. The trendy restaurant is a hub for pure, raw superfoods, cold-pressed juices, smoothies, and coffee. Daluma's offerings are 100% organic and beautiful to look at, too.

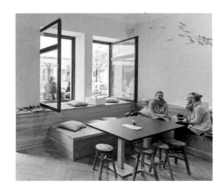

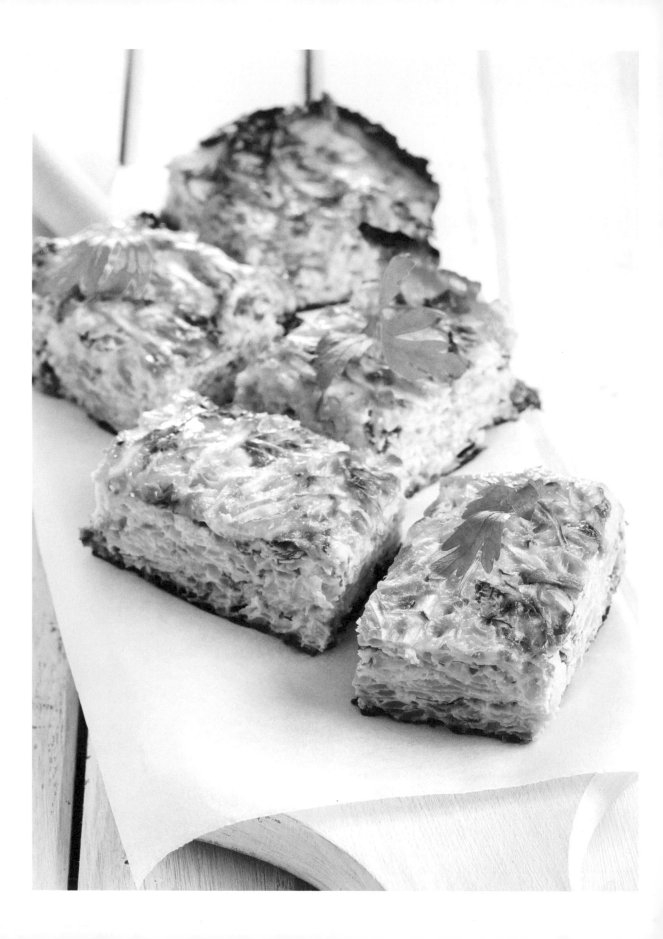

REBECCA VALLANCE
ZUCCHINI SLICE

PREPARATION

1) Preheat oven to 340°F / 170°C. Grease and line a 12 x 8 in. / 30 x 20 cm pan.

2) Beat eggs in a large bowl until combined.

3) Add flour and beat until smooth, then add zucchini, onion, bacon, cheese, and oil, then stir to combine.

4) Pour into the prepared pan and bake in oven for 30 minutes or until cooked through.

5) Serve with a green salad.

INGREDIENTS

» 5 eggs
» 1 ¼ cups / 150 g gluten-free flour (sifted)
» 2 cups / 375 g zucchini (grated)
» 1 large onion (diced)
» 7 oz / 200 g rindless bacon (diced)
» 1 cup / 115 g cheddar cheese (grated)
» 4 ½ tbsp olive oil
» Green salad to serve

REBECCA VALLANCE

Since showing her label at New York Fashion Week, Australian fashion designer Rebecca Vallance has firmly established herself as one to watch on the international scene. She has become one of Australia's latest fashion exports and a favorite amongst style icons, celebrities, and top models around the globe. Here she shares a beloved dish she usually cooks for her son.

www.rebeccavallance.com

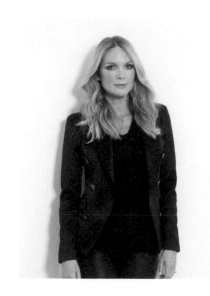

LORNA JANE
SEAFOOD PAELLA

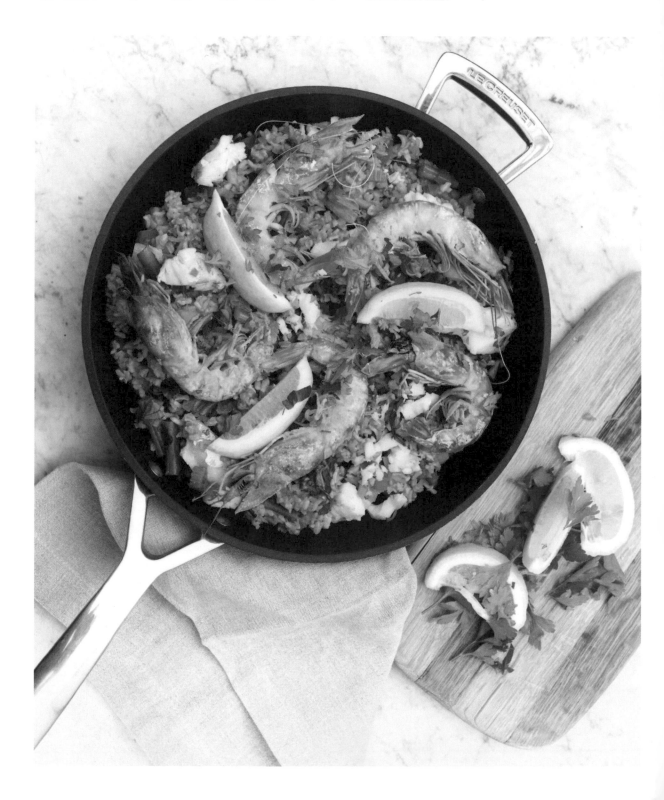

PREPARATION

1) Heat oil in a medium deep frying pan. Cook onion and garlic, stirring, until onion softens.

2) Add celery, bell pepper, fennel, cumin, paprika, and tomato paste; cook, stirring until vegetables are tender. Add rice, saffron, and bay leaf; stir to coat rice in vegetable mixture. Add tomatoes and 1 cup / 240 ml of water; cook, stirring, until liquid is absorbed. Add remaining water and tamari; cook, covered, over medium-low heat, stirring occasionally for about 45 minutes or until liquid is absorbed and rice is tender.

3) Stir beans and spinach into rice mixture. Top with fish, prawns, and scallops. Cook, covered, for about 5 minutes or until seafood is just cooked through. Season to taste.

4) Cover paella and let stand for 5 minutes.

5) Sprinkle paella with parsley. Serve with lemon wedges.

INGREDIENTS

» 1 tbsp cold-pressed extra-virgin coconut oil
» 1 small red onion (chopped finely)
» 3 garlic cloves (crushed)
» 2 stalks celery (trimmed and diced)
» 1 medium bell pepper (diced)
» 1 tsp each ground fennel, ground cumin, and paprika
» 2 tbsp tomato paste
» 1 cup / 200 g brown short-grain rice
» Pinch of saffron threads
» 1 bay leaf
» 3 medium tomatoes (chopped coarsely)
» 2 cups / 480 ml filtered water
» 1 tbsp tamari
» ¾ cup / 75 g green beans (trimmed and chopped coarsely)
» 1 cup / 30 g baby spinach leaves
» 11 oz / 300 g firm white fish fillets (cut into 2-in. / 5 cm pieces)
» 6 uncooked medium king prawns or shrimps (shelled, deveined, tails intact)
» 6 scallops (roe removed)
» Salt and pepper to taste
» ¼ cup / 5 g loosely packed fresh flat-leaf parsley leaves
» 1 lemon (cut into wedges)

LORNA JANE

Active living advocate, business entrepreneur, fashion designer, and author, Lorna Jane Clarkson is the founder and Chief Creative Officer of multi-award-winning activewear label, Lorna Jane. She is renowned for her active living philosophy which inspires women to live their best life, through the daily practice of her principles: move, nourish, believe.

www.lornajane.com

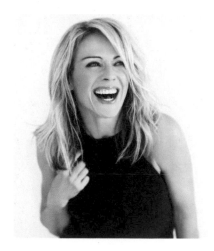

LIORA BELS
ROASTED BEETS & PARSNIPS WITH BEET HORSERADISH CASHEW CREAM

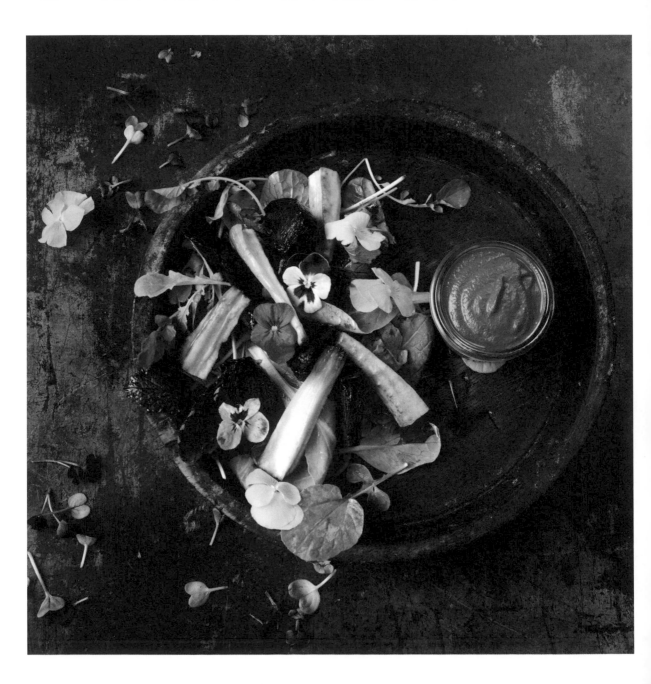

PREPARATION

Roasted Beets and Parsnips:

1) Preheat the oven to 350°F / 180°C.

2) Prepare the beets and parsnips by placing them into a baking dish, drizzle with coconut oil, and add a pinch of salt.

3) Bake for 30 minutes or until soft and juicy. Then change to grill, increase to 390°F / 200°C and roast for another 10 minutes or until slightly brown. Let cool and serve lukewarm.

Beet Horseradish Cream:

1) Blend all ingredients in your high-speed blender until smooth.

2) Add more salt and horseradish if you desire a stronger taste and repeat the blending procedure.

Dressing:

1) Mix lemon juice, olive oil, and salt.

To Serve:

1) Place herbs and salad in a bowl. Mix well with the dressing.

2) Place parsnips and beets on top of the salad, sprinkle with daikon cress and serve with beet horseradish cashew cream.

LIORA BELS

Liora Bels is a health food chef, author, certified nutrition expert, as well as a food and style consultant. She is passionate about inspiring and educating people about the art of eating well and consults for clients in the gastronomy, design, health, sports, and travel sectors. During her worldwide travels and time spent living abroad, Liora gained valuable insights and cultivated her fascination with nutrition and health food. Liora's philosophy is rooted in a holistic approach. Not only does she believe in the healing benefits of plant-based, wholesome nutrition, but also that a conscious lifestyle has a positive impact on our overall well-being and a better future.

www.liorabels.com

INGREDIENTS

Roasted Beets and Parsnips:
- » *6 small parsnips (quartered)*
- » *2 large beets (quartered)*
- » *1 large tbsp cold-pressed coconut oil*
- » *Pinch of salt (Maldon or Himalayan pink salt)*

Beet Horseradish Cream:
- » *¾ cup / 180–200 ml filtered water*
- » *2 cups / 250 g cashews (soaked for 6 hours in filtered water and washed thoroughly)*
- » *1 large beet*
- » *Juice of 1 lemon*
- » *3 ⅓ tbsp fresh horseradish*
- » *Salt to taste (Maldon or Himalayan pink salt)*

Dressing:
- » *Juice of 1 lemon*
- » *4 tbsp cold-pressed olive oil*
- » *Pinch of salt (Maldon or Himalayan pink salt)*

Salad:
- » *¼ cup / 10 g fresh mint leaves*
- » *2 heaping cups / 90 g fresh parsley (roughly chopped)*
- » *4 cups / 140 g wild herb and baby leaf salad*
- » *A handful of daikon cress*

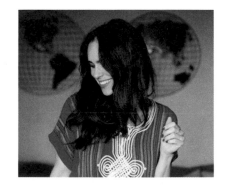

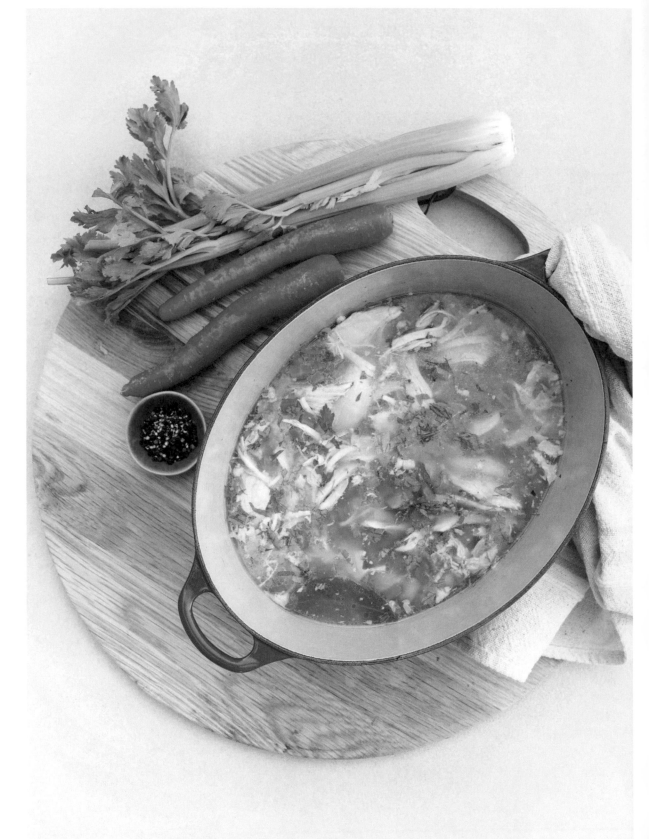

CHRISTIANE DUIGAN
SLOW COOKED CHICKEN SOUP

PREPARATION

1) Sauté the carrot, celery, onion, and garlic in a large cooking pot that can be sealed.

2) Place the chicken into the pot and fill with filtered water.

3) Season with salt and pepper, add herbs and vinegar.

4) Cover and cook on 210°F / 100°C in the oven for 4–6 hours or on the stove top on the lowest setting for the same amount of time.

5) To serve: The chicken will easily break into pieces. I like to serve it lightly separated with a teaspoon of butter and extra freshly ground black pepper. If you have the patience, however, you can remove all the bones from the chicken once it has cooled down. If you put less water, the dish will be like a yummy chicken stew! Serve it with sweet potato mash for a heartier, wintry meal.

INGREDIENTS

» *1 whole chicken*
» *2 carrots (finely diced)*
» *1 stalk celery (finely diced)*
» *1 small yellow onion (diced)*
» *3–4 garlic cloves (roughly chopped)*
» *2 bay leaves*
» *4 sprigs fresh thyme*
» *2 tbsp apple cider vinegar*
» *A small handful of sea salt*
» *Plenty of freshly ground black pepper*
» *Butter to serve*

CHRISTIANE DUIGAN

Christiane Duigan is the Clean & Lean book's very own cover girl, a busy mom of two and the wife of Bodyism and Clean & Lean founder James Duigan. A regular jet-setter, Christiane travels the world in the name of Bodyism to feel inspired by the latest innovations in fashion and health trends. "Positivity always shines through and beauty comes from within," Christiane says, "but how you dress plays such a huge part in how you feel. Love yourself, love others and love life."

www.aus.cleanandlean.com
www.bodyism.com

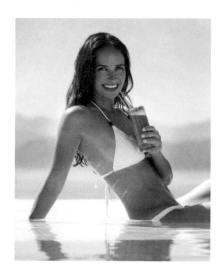

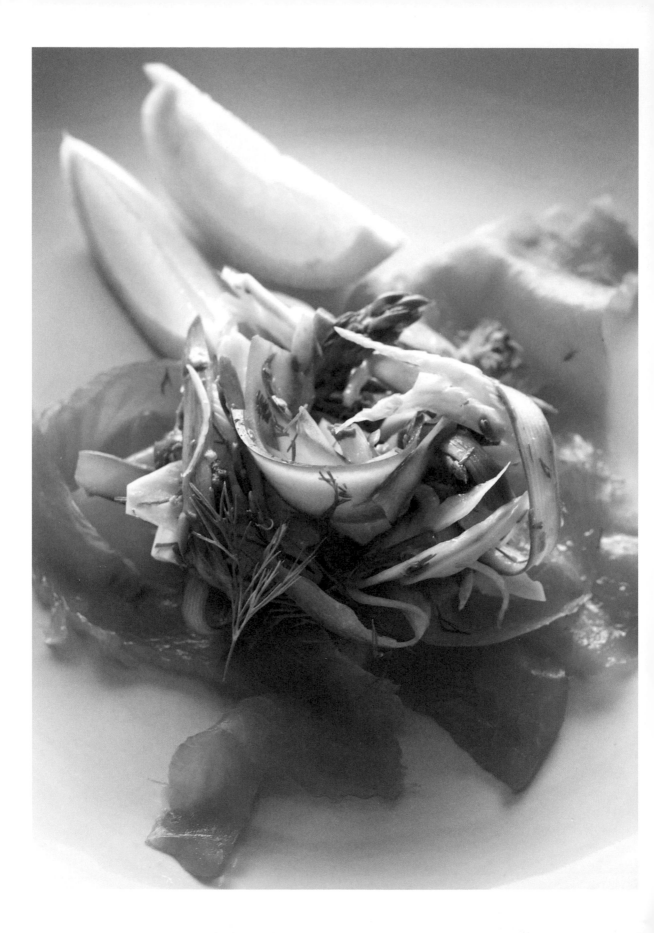

TALI SHINE
SMOKED SALMON & GREEN SALAD

PREPARATION

1) Arrange the smoked or poached salmon slices onto plates.

2) Using a vegetable peeler, slice the fennel, cucumber, and asparagus lengthways into thin slices.

3) Place in a bowl with the capers and dill.

4) Drizzle oil, vinegar, and lemon juice and gently toss.

5) Place the salad on top of salmon slices. Season with rock salt, pepper, and lemon slices.

INGREDIENTS

» *1 lb / 500 g smoked or poached salmon*
» *4 tbsp lemon juice*
» *1 lemon (sliced)*
» *1 tbsp rinsed capers*
» *1 tsp dill (finely chopped)*
» *1 ½ tbsp extra-virgin olive oil*
» *1 tsp apple cider vinegar*
» *2 bunches of asparagus*
» *1 large fennel plant*
» *1 cucumber*
» *Rock salt and pepper to taste*

TALI SAYS:

"Wild-caught smoked salmon is filled with omegas that make skin glow and hair shine. The greens in this salad, particularly the fennel and asparagus, are filled with nutrients and are wonderful digestive aids."

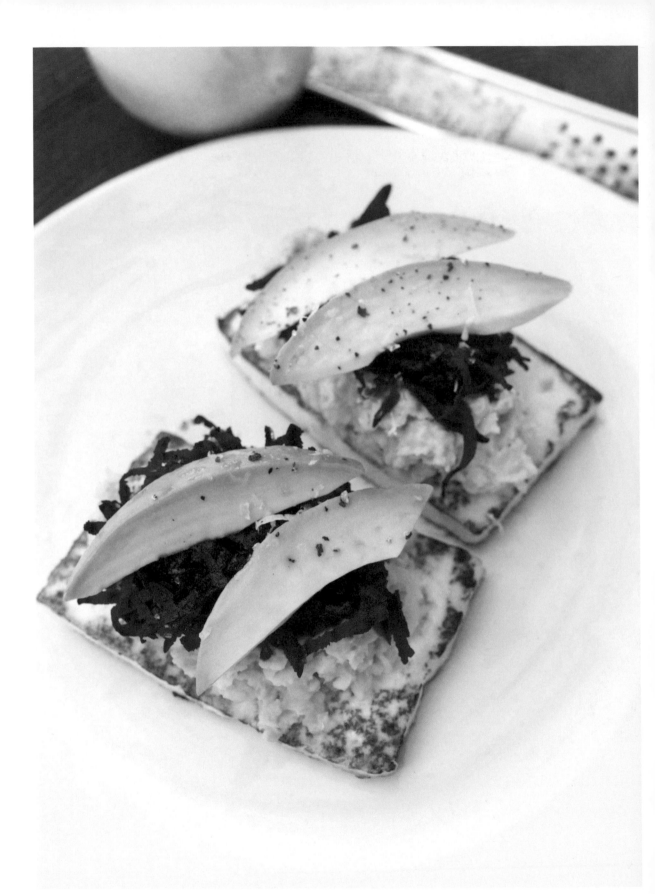

RACHAEL FINCH
TOFU, HUMMUS, &
BEET STACK

PREPARATION

1) In large mixing bowl, add chickpeas, 1 tablespoon olive oil, lemon juice, salt, and pepper. Mash until thick and chunky.

2) Season tofu and cook on medium heat in oil for a minute or so on all sides (I like mine nice and crispy!).

3) Serve by building a stack: tofu patty, spoonful of hummus, beet, and avocado slices.

INGREDIENTS

» *2 x 3.5 oz / 2 x 100 g squares of firm tofu*
» *½ beet (skin removed and grated)*
» *1 can of chickpeas (washed)*
» *Juice from a large wedge of lemon*
» *2 tbsp olive oil*
» *Salt and pepper to taste*
» *Avocado slices for garnish*

RACHAEL FINCH

Rachael Finch is a woman of many titles. The Australian beauty pageant titleholder, television reporter, model, media personality, and brand ambassador has always been conscious about taking care of her body and living a wholesome, holistic lifestyle.

www.rachaelfinch.com

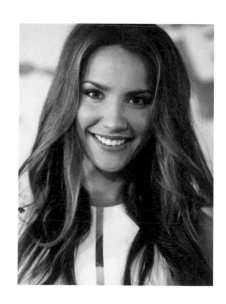

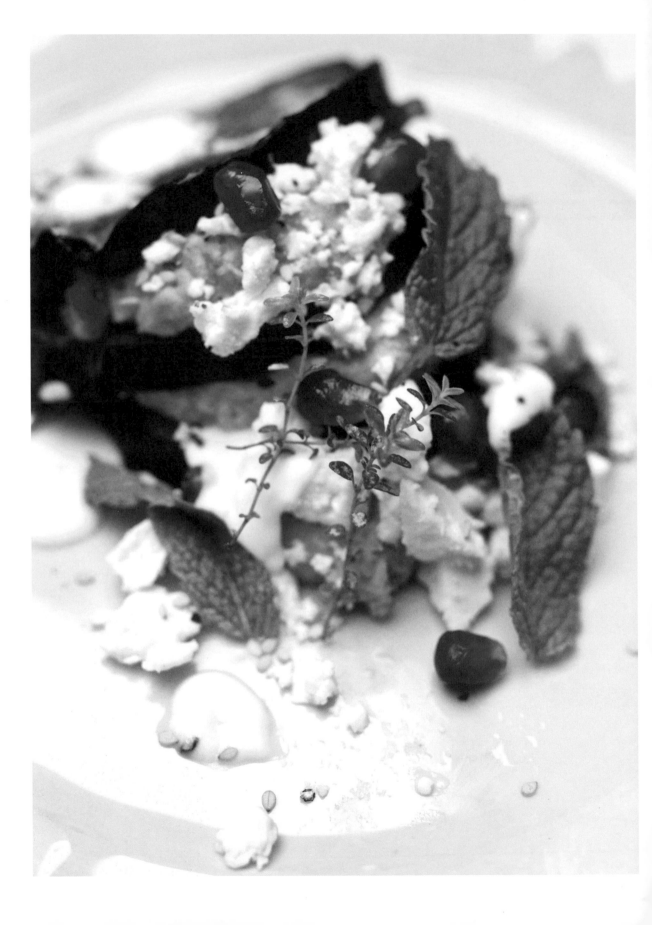

GRACE BELGRAVIA
ROASTED MEDITERRANEAN SALAD

PREPARATION

1) To make the hummus, start by drizzling the bell pepper with 1 tablespoon of rapeseed oil, season and roast at 390°F / 200°C for about 30–40 minutes until soft and the skin has started to turn black. Put in a bowl and cover with cling wrap.

2) Cut the eggplant into 4 thick slices, about 2 in. / 5 cm. Drizzle with 3 tablespoons of rapeseed oil, season, and sprinkle with thyme. Roast at 350°F / 180°C for about 30 minutes until cooked. After 15 minutes, add a little extra oil if the eggplant looks dry.

3) To finish the hummus, peel the skin off of the cooled bell pepper and remove all seeds.

4) Put the bell pepper into a food processor and blitz with the juice of half a lemon, olive oil, chickpeas, tahini, grated garlic, paprika, and dried chili flakes (if you like heat). Season to taste.

5) For the dressing, mix the kefir with the juice from the other lemon half and season as desired with salt and black pepper.

6) To serve, spoon hummus on the plate, place 2 pieces of eggplant on top, crumble over feta, drizzle with kefir dressing, and sprinkle with pomegranate seeds, mint leaves, and sesame seeds.

Note: Vegans can simply remove the cheese and use coconut yogurt for the dressing. Equally delicious!

INGREDIENTS

(Serves 2)

- » *1 red bell pepper*
- » *4 tbsp rapeseed oil*
- » *2 large eggplants*
- » *1 lemon thyme sprig*
- » *¾ cup and 1 tbsp / 200 g chickpeas (cooked)*
- » *2 tbsp tahini*
- » *Juice of 1 lemon*
- » *1 tbsp extra-virgin olive oil*
- » *1 tbsp smoked paprika*
- » *1 small garlic clove (grated)*
- » *1 sprinkle dried chili flakes (optional)*
- » *4 tbsp kefir*
- » *½ cup / 100 g Greek feta cheese*
- » *1 small bunch of fresh mint*
- » *⅓ cup / 50 g pomegranate seeds*
- » *1 tbsp sesame seeds (optional)*
- » *Sea salt and black pepper*

GRACE BELGRAVIA

Grace Belgravia is a health, well-being, and lifestyle members club for women in London. The club mantra is to be inspired, empowered, and rejuvenated—no matter what your age. The club champions preventative medicine and aging well, so people can feel the very best they can be.

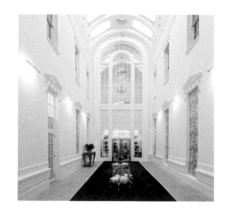

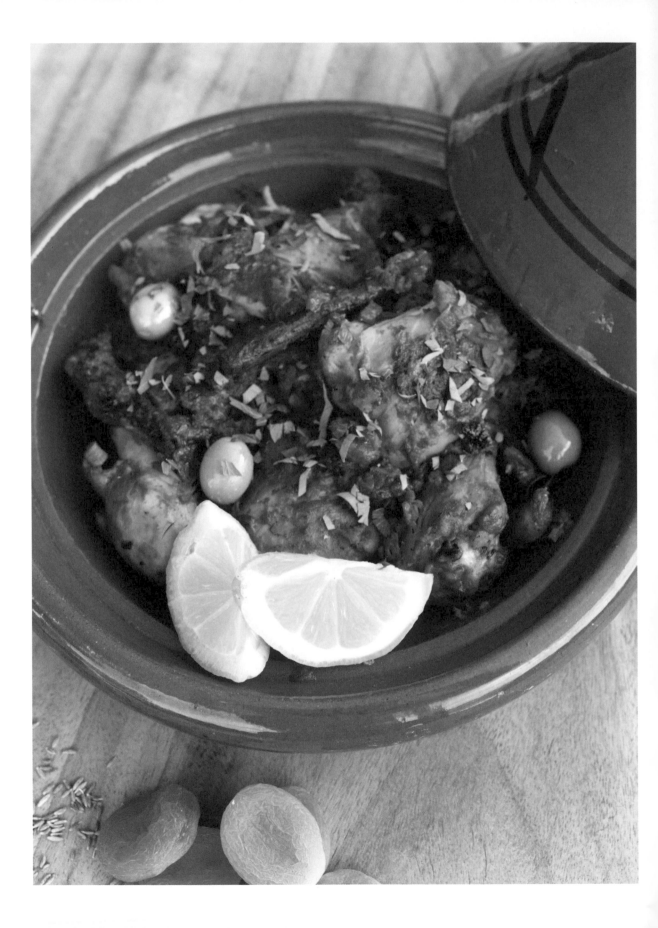

ALIYA HOLLAND
SAFFRON APRICOT CHICKEN

PREPARATION

1) Preheat oven to 350°F / 180°C.
2) Place a pinch of saffron in a small bowl and cover with warm stock.
3) In a casserole pan, sweat the onions with the ginger and garlic, add the spices, tomatoes and everything else (except the chicken, sliced almonds, and fresh herbs). Simmer for 15–20 minutes.
4) In a shallow pan, brown the chicken pieces and put aside in a baking/tagine dish.
5) Pour the sauce over the chicken and bake in a tagine or in a baking dish covered in foil for 40 minutes.
6) Take the foil off and continue to oven roast for 10–15 minutes longer to get a more caramelized finish.
7) Dress with fresh herbs and toasted sliced almonds.
8) Serve with a crisp green salad, on its own, or with steamed quinoa for a hungrier crowd!

INGREDIENTS

(Serves 4)
» 8 skinless chicken pieces (thighs work well)
» 2 tbsp olive oil
» 1 large onion (finely chopped)
» 2 tsp garlic (finely chopped)
» Thumb-sized piece ginger (minced)
» 2 tsp ground Moroccan Spice (or 1 tsp cumin, 1 tsp cilantro)
» 1 cinnamon stick
» 14 oz / 400 g canned chopped tomatoes
» 1 tbsp runny honey
» Large pinch of saffron
» 1 ¼ cups / 300 ml hot chicken stock
» ½ preserved lemon (finely chopped)
» ½ cup / 100 g dried apricots
» 1 handful of green queen olives
» ⅓ cup / 25 g sliced almonds (toasted)
» 2 tbsp cilantro and 2 tbsp flat-leaf parsley (roughly chopped)

ALIYA HOLLAND

Aliya is a naturopath and nutritional therapist living in Cape Town who just loves her food. Her Middle Eastern and Scandinavian heritage has infused a mixture of complex aromatic flavors and combined it with simplicity. She specializes in working with families and individuals to get the most out of their nutrition without any compromise on taste or enjoyment. Her ethos centers on family cooking and eating together, enjoying the same healthy and fresh food. When she is not in the kitchen, Aliya is out and about sharing her knowledge, writing articles on wellness and nutrition, and motivating her friends and wider circle to live, eat, and move better. She is also a self-confessed tahini addict.

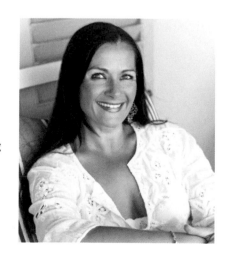

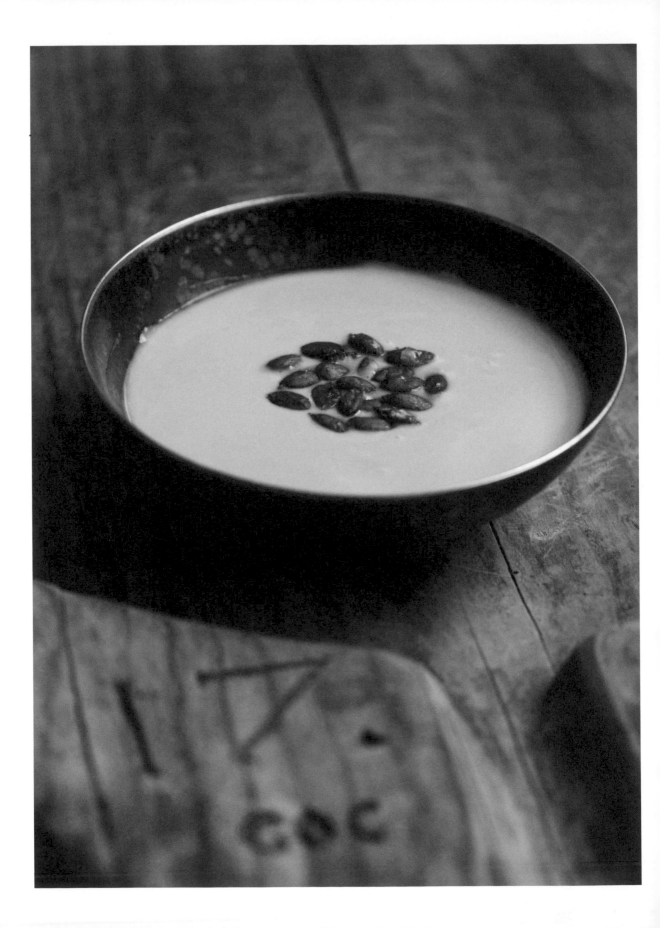

GLOW HEALTHBAR
SPICE ME UP BUTTERNUT SQUASH SOUP

PREPARATION

This soup is featured in all of Glow's cleanse programs. It's packed with vitamin A, fiber-rich celery, and flavorful curry powder.

1) Preheat oven to 350°F / 180°C.
2) Roughly chop butternut squash, place onto a baking tray with a drizzle of olive oil or coconut oil and season with Himalayan pink salt.
3) Repeat the same process with the celery and onion.
4) Place on separate trays in the oven.
5) Take out once you can pierce squash with a fork and it is nice and soft.
6) Place into a blender and mix in the curry, bouillon, coconut mousse, coconut oil, and ginger.
7) Add the coconut water and regular water.
8) Blend until smooth and creamy.

INGREDIENTS

» 1 ⅛ cups / 500 g butternut squash
» Olive oil (or coconut oil) for seasoning
» 1 onion (roughly chopped)
» ½ cup / 40 g celery (roughly chopped)
» 2 tbsp coconut mousse
» Thumb-sized piece ginger
» 1 tsp curry powder
» 1 tbsp coconut oil
» 1 tsp vegetable bouillon
» 1 ⅔ cups / 400 ml water
» 1 ½ cups / 360 ml coconut water
» Himalayan pink salt

GLOW HEALTHBAR

Glow Healthbar, located in the idyllic mountain village of Gstaad, is the area's go-to place for healthy juices, soups, snacks, and superfoods. Glow was opened in 2013 by friends Diana D'Hendecourt and Blanca Brillembourg who longed for the fresh cold-press juices they found in New York and Miami. Blanca's daughter, Princess Tatiana Blatnik, is also an active contributor to their menus. Tatiana has inherited her mother's passion for all things healthy and feels most at home researching and trying different recipes.

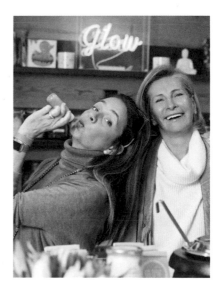

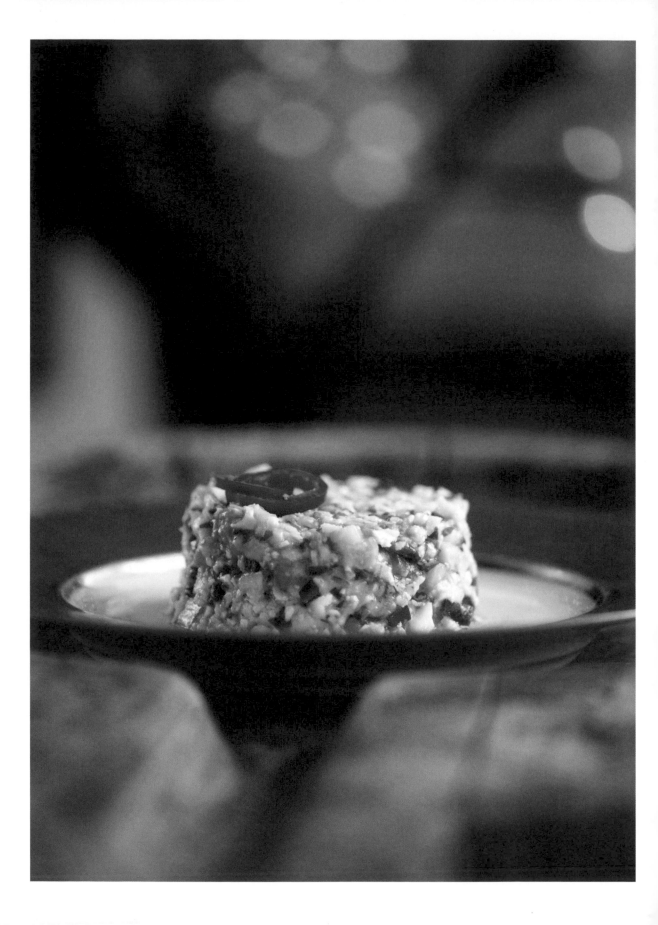

GLOW HEALTHBAR
DETOX CAULIFLOWER "TABBOULEH"

PREPARATION

1) Shave the cauliflower with a sharp knife (or high-speed food processor) into small "rice" pieces.

2) Roughly chop the parsley.

3) Dice cucumber into very small pieces.

4) Cut chili in half, scrape out seeds, and chop into very small pieces.

5) Cut avocado into small cubes.

6) Throw all ingredients into a bowl and add lemon juice, olive oil, and Himalayan pink salt to taste.

Note: For a sweeter version, drizzle honey into the mixture.

INGREDIENTS

» ⅝ cup / 200 g cauliflower
» 4.8 lbs / 2.2 kg cucumber
» 1 avocado
» 2 ⅓ cups / 60 g parsley
» 5 oz / 150 g chili
» Juice of 1 lemon
» 5 tbsp olive oil
» ½ tsp Himalayan pink salt to taste

HRH PRINCESS TATIANA SAYS:

"This is one of my favorite recipes. It is easy to make, crunchy, fresh, alkaline, and grain-free! A great snack, meal, or side dish, this Detox Cauliflower 'Tabbouleh' is a versatile dish you can have at home, at the office, or even on a flight. Play around with what you add to make it your own—and enjoy!"

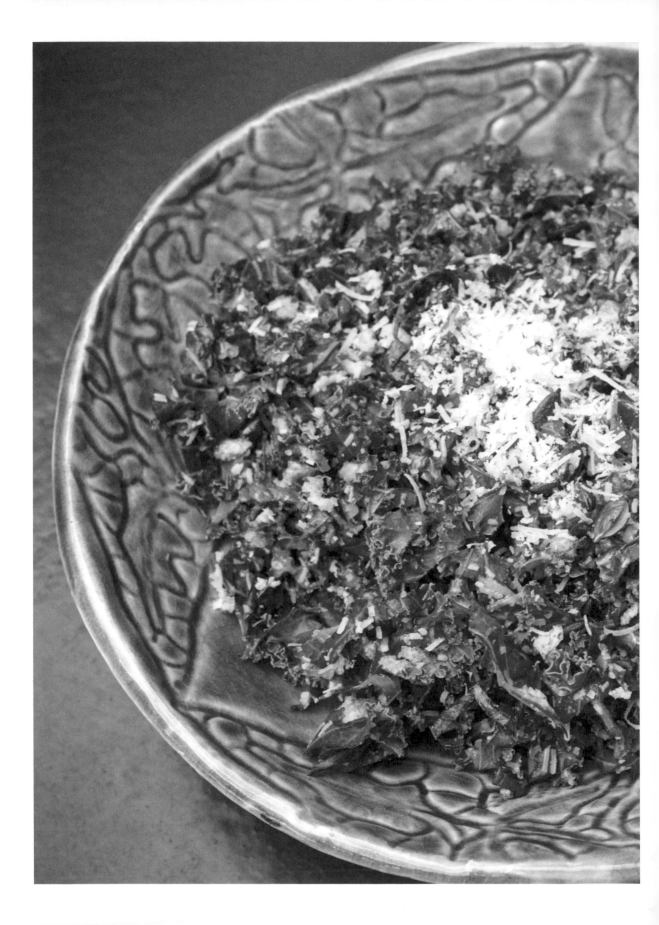

GABRIELA PEACOCK
TUSCAN KALE SALAD

PREPARATION

1) Trim the bottom off the kale stems. Slice the kale into ¾-in. / 2 cm ribbons. Place the kale in a large bowl.

2) Toast the gluten-free bread until golden brown on both sides and dry throughout. Tear into small pieces and pulse in a food processor until the mixture forms coarse crumbs.

3) Lightly toast pumpkin seeds using a small amount of coconut oil.

4) Place minced garlic in a small bowl. Add cheese, 3 tablespoons olive oil, lemon juice, pinch of salt, pepper flakes, and black pepper. Whisk to combine.

5) Pour dressing over kale and toss well.

6) Top with the bread crumbs, pumpkin seeds, additional cheese, and a drizzle of oil.

INGREDIENTS

» *1 bunch of kale*
» *2 thin slices gluten-free bread*
» *½ garlic clove (minced)*
» *¼ tsp ground rock salt*
» *¼ cup / 25 g (or small handful) pecorino cheese (grated)*
» *3 tbsp extra-virgin olive oil*
» *Juice of 1 lemon*
» *⅛ tsp red pepper flakes*
» *Freshly ground black pepper to taste*
» *Handful of pumpkin seeds*
» *Coconut oil*

GABRIELA PEACOCK

Former model Gabriela Peacock is London's go-to nutritionalist for the smart set. Her celebrity clientele includes members of the young royal family, high-profile business leaders, television presenters, and international models. She is also an avid kaleologist. Gabriela has recently launched her own range of supplements, Gabriela Peacock Nutrition.

www.gpnutrition.co.uk

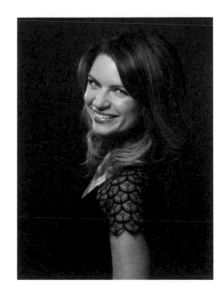

PAN SEARED LOCAL FISH

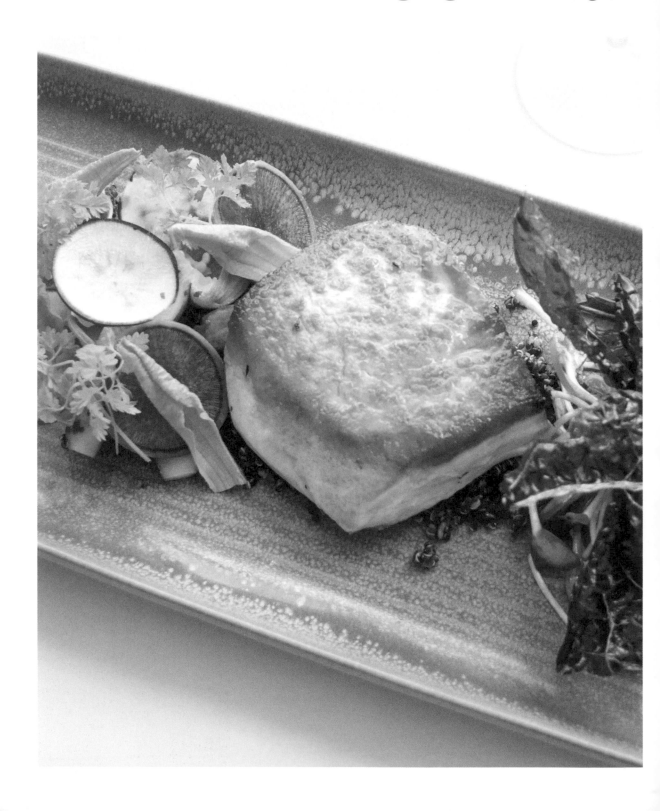

PREPARATION

1) Place quinoa in to a medium sized pot add 2 tablespoons of rice bran oil. Toast until lightly brown.

2) Add 2 cups / 480 ml of water and cook on low heat until water has absorbed, about 10–12 minutes.

3) Set aside and allow to sit for 10 minutes before serving.

4) Remove pollen from inside the zucchini flower and slice the whole thing in half. Set aside.

5) Set up a steaming pot ready to cook the flowers (they will not take long to cook).

6) To prepare the salad, wash sprouts and herbs then put in ice water. Slice radish as fine as possible and place into ice water.

7) Dry salad well on a towel or use a salad spinner to remove excess water.

8) To prepare lemon dressing, zest lemons into the sprout salad mix, place juice into a bowl. Add 2 tablespoons good olive oil, a pinch of salt, and a splash of nice vinegar.

9) Place fish onto a piece of kitchen paper to get rid of any excess water.

10) Place a heavy base frypan over low heat. Once the pan is hot, pour 2–3 tablespoons of rice bran oil or coconut oil into the pan. The oil should start to smoke a little—this is very important!

11) Sprinkle fish with sea salt flakes and gently place down into the pan. The fish should start to sizzle instantly.

12) Leave on a medium to high heat for 3 minutes, watching to see the flesh or skin turn a beautiful golden color. Do not move the pan or fish until you see this happening.

13) Turn fish over with a spatula and place into an oven (preheat to 350°F / 180°C) or turn pan to a low heat and allow to cook for a further 3–4 minutes depending on the size of the fish fillet.

14) Serve fish with the salad.

INGREDIENTS

» 5.5–6.5 oz / 160–180 g portion of fish
» 2 zucchini flowers
» Sprouts (sunflower sprouts, alfalfa or any other sprout available)
» 1 bunch of red radish
» Juice and zest of 2 large lemons
» Chervil, parsley, fennel, or other herbs (pick nice leaves)
» Kale leaves
» 1 cup / 170 g quinoa, red or white
» Rice bran oil (or coconut oil)
» Olive oil
» Vinegar

Note: When checking to see if the fish is cooked, you can test it by using a toothpick and slide it into the flesh. If it goes through without too much resistance, take fish out of the pan and rest for 2 minutes. You can also place a skewer into the thickest part of the fish. Let it sit for 5 seconds. Pull it out and touch the skewer to the back of your hand. If it's warm to hot, the fish is cooked perfectly. Take out and rest for 2 minutes.

RAE'S ON WATEGOS

Rae's on Wategos is an exclusive boutique retreat in a luxurious beachfront setting. Its elegant restaurant offers modern Australian cuisine in a secluded corner of Byron Bay. The restaurant's 50 seat al fresco dining space makes this eatery one of Australia's best.

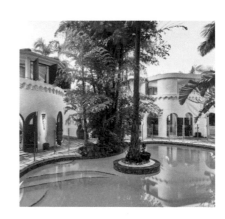

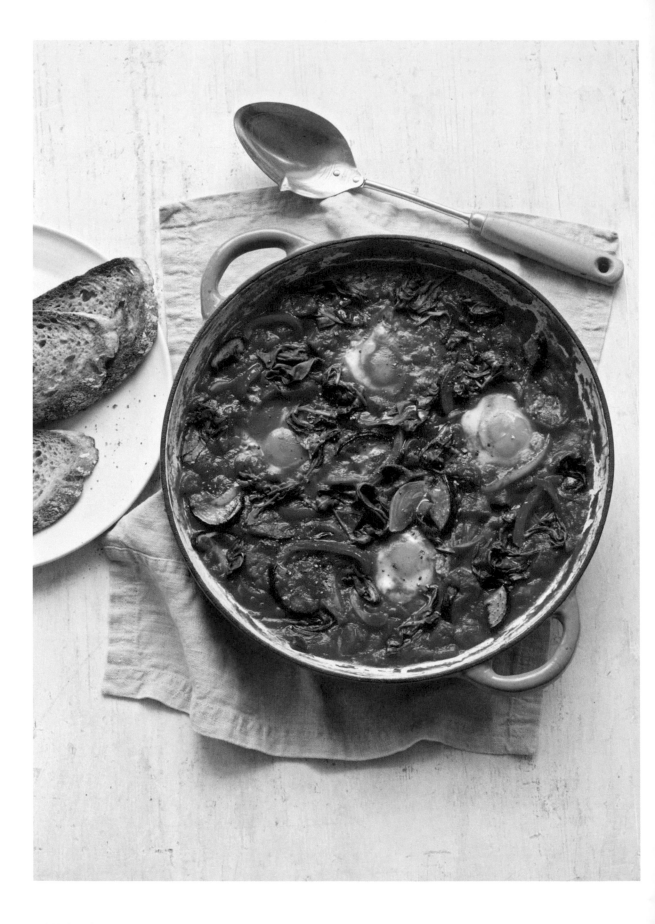

JAMES DUIGAN
SHAKSHUKA

PREPARATION

1) Put a deep, large lidded frying pan or skillet over a high heat and melt the coconut oil. Add the onion and sauté for a few minutes until softened. Add garlic and stir.

2) After a few minutes, add the spices and tomato purée and stir. Add the eggplant and peppers and leave to soften, stirring every couple of minutes.

3) Add the chopped tomatoes and stir. Mix in the fresh cilantro and parsley and continue to cook for 10–15 minutes. Season to taste.

4) Using a big spoon, make 4 small wells in each quarter of the mixture to pour the eggs into. Try to pour them in as quickly as you can so that they all have roughly the same cooking time. Cover the pan with the lid and leave the eggs to cook for roughly 3 minutes (make sure you don't overcook them as the runny yolk is the best bit).

5) Just before the eggs are cooked, scatter the spinach over the top, put the lid back on and leave it to wilt for about 30 seconds. Season with salt and pepper and serve. We love to serve this with a spoonful of Greek yogurt or tahini as well and a sprinkling of fresh cilantro.

INGREDIENTS

» 1 onion (diced)
» 2 garlic cloves (crushed)
» 1 tsp ground cumin
» 1 tsp mild chili powder
» 1 tsp paprika
» 1 tbsp tomato purée
» 1 eggplant (sliced widthwise)
» 1 red bell pepper (cut into strips)
» 1 yellow bell pepper (cut into strips)
» 14 oz / 400 g canned chopped tomatoes
» 1 tbsp fresh cilantro (chopped), plus extra for garnish
» 1 tbsp fresh parsley (chopped)
» 4 eggs
» 2 ⅓ cups / 70 g spinach
» Sea salt and freshly ground black pepper
» Coconut oil, for frying
» Greek yogurt or tahini (optional)

JAMES DUIGAN

Ten years ago, James Duigan made it his mission to empower as many people as possible by spreading his Clean & Lean philosophy. He wanted people from all walks of life to realize their physical and mental potential so that they could experience a happier and healthier life. After qualifying as a trainer, James soon began working with supermodel Elle Macpherson and very quickly acquired a glittering list of celebrity clientele including Emilia Clarke, Hugh Grant, and Lara Stone. James recognized that his clients weren't achieving their potential due to the stresses of their fast-paced lives, and soon Clean & Lean was born. He made it his mission to create a range of supplements, recipe books, and teas that would enable people all over the world to live a clean, healthy life with less fuss.

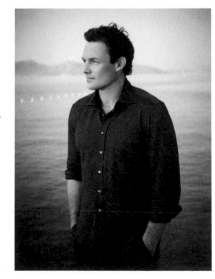

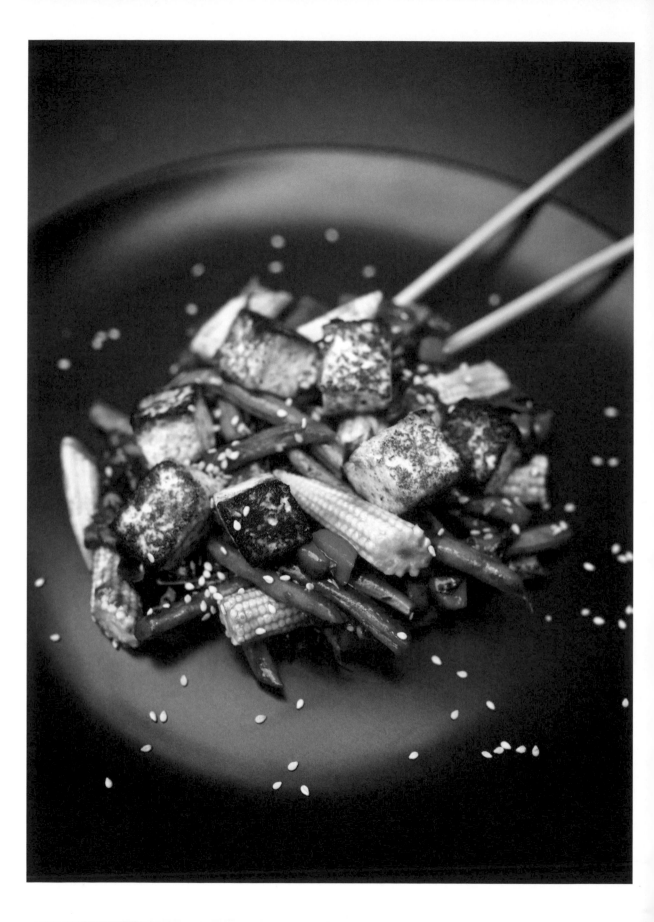

DANAI KOUGIOULI
VEGAN TOFU STIR FRY

PREPARATION

1) Preheat oven to 400°F / 200°C.
2) Remove tofu from package. Drain and place it between two thick paper towels. Then place a plate or bowl on top along with something heavy like a book.
3) Let it dry for about 15 minutes, changing your paper towels if they get too wet. Slice tofu into cubes.
4) Arrange tofu on a baking sheet and bake for a total of 30–35 minutes, flipping once halfway through to ensure even cooking.
5) Once it's golden brown and a bit firm, remove from the oven and set it out to dry.
6) In a small mixing bowl, whisk together all of the sauce ingredients. Set aside.
7) Place pan on medium heat, add sesame oil. Next add veggies and toss to coat.
8) Cook for 5–7 minutes, stirring often. When the vegetables are softened and have some color, add the sauce and stir. Then add the tofu and stir for another 3–5 minutes.
9) Serve over brown rice.

INGREDIENTS

Tofu and Vegetables:
- » *1 medium package firm or extra firm tofu*
- » *1 cup / 150 g green beans (chopped)*
- » *1 cup / 150 g carrots (diced)*
- » *1 cup / 300 g baby corns*
- » *1 cup / 70 g kale (chopped)*
- » *2 tbsp toasted sesame oil (or peanut or coconut)*

Sauce:
- » *¼ cup / 60 ml low-sodium, gluten-free tamari soy sauce*
- » *1 tbsp fresh ginger (grated)*
- » *2 tbsp brown sugar (or coconut sugar)*
- » *1 tbsp agave nectar*

Garnish:
- » *Brown rice to taste*

DANAI KOUGIOULI

Born and raised in Greece, Danai Kougiouli is one of London's and New York's most sought after prenatal and Jivamukti yoga teachers. A former competitive runner, Danai was first introduced to yoga in her teens as a means of improving breathing, focus, and confidence for competition. Today, her classes are filled with London's fashion elite, tastemakers, and celebrities including Sienna Miller, Thandi Newton, and Aaron Taylor-Johnson. Danai follows a vegan diet and believes fashion and taste don't need to be compromised due to healthy lifestyle choices.

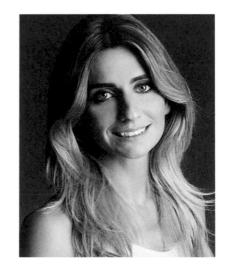

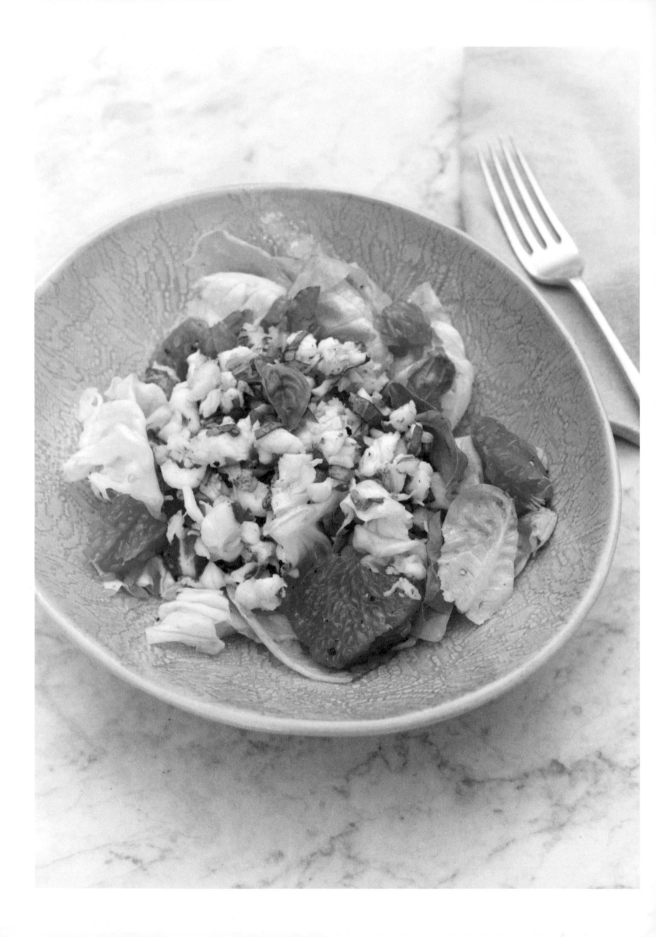

MILTON PARK
CRAB CHILI & PINK GRAPEFRUIT SALAD

PREPARATION

1) Top and tail the grapefruits. Stand them on one of the flat ends and carefully trim off the skin with a knife, turning the fruit as you go. To segment them, follow the white lines with your knife and gently twist the knife out to remove each segment.

2) Place the segments in a bowl and squeeze all the juice from the center parts on top.

3) Pick through the crab meat and remove any bits of shell. Place in a separate bowl with the chilis.

4) Tear apart most of the basil leaves, then spoon over 2 table-spoons of the grapefruit juice and add 4 teaspoons of extra-virgin olive oil. Season with a little bit of pink salt and a pinch of pepper. Gently mix together.

5) Add the salad leaves to the bowl with the grapefruit segments, add a lug of extra-virgin olive oil, a pinch of salt and pepper, then toss to coat each leaf.

6) Arrange the salad over four plates, top with the grapefruit segments from the bottom of the bowl, followed by equal amounts of the dressed crab.

7) Finish by garnishing with the reserved basil leaves.

INGREDIENTS

(Serves 4)

» *2 pink grapefruits*
» *1 heaping cup / 200 g white crab meat from sustainable sources (ask your local fishmonger)*
» *2 fresh red chilies (deseeded and finely chopped)*
» *1 bunch of fresh basil leaves (chopped), and some for reserve*
» *Extra-virgin olive oil*
» *Himalayan pink salt*
» *Freshly ground black pepper*
» *1 head of fresh butter lettuce, (ripped into bite size pieces, washed and spun dry)*

MILTON PARK

Set on its own beautiful, secluded hilltop, Milton Park Country House Hotel & Spa is a five-star hotel offering luxurious accommodation, fine cuisine, and impeccable yet discreet service in an atmosphere of relaxed sophistication. This escape in the Southern Highlands of New South Wales was established at the turn of the 20th century by the Hordern Family of retail and pastoral fame. Guests are stunned by breathtaking views to the horizon in every direction over some of Australia's best gardens.

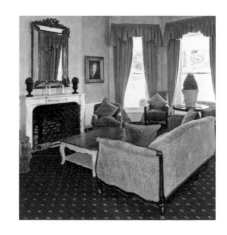

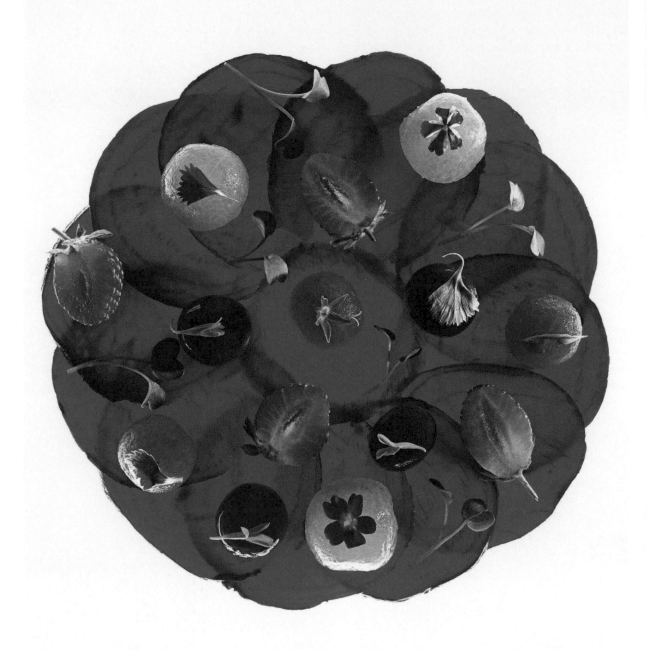

HOTEL ARTS BARCELONA
BEET CARPACCIO

PREPARATION

1) To start, cut the cooked beets into very thin slices (0.04–0.08 in. / 1–2 mm).

2) Decorate with the tomatoes, strawberries, and the black olives spheres.

3) To finish, add arugula leaves, sprouts, flowers, and balsamic vinegar reduction.

INGREDIENTS

» *35 oz / 1 kg beets (cooked)*
» *Red cherry tomatoes (peeled)*
» *Yellow cherry tomatoes (peeled)*
» *Black olive spheres*
» *Strawberries (halved)*
» *7 oz / 200 g arugula leaves*
» *Sprouts and flowers to garnish*
» *Balsamic vinegar reduction to taste*
» *Olive oil to taste*

HOTEL ARTS BARCELONA

One of the Mediterranean's most blissful retreats, Hotel Arts Barcelona is a place where exceptional service comes as standard. The cultural hub offers six restaurants and bars, including the two Michelin-star Enoteca, making it a premiere fine dining destination whether you're hungry for an informal breakfast or haute cuisine.

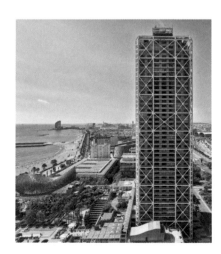

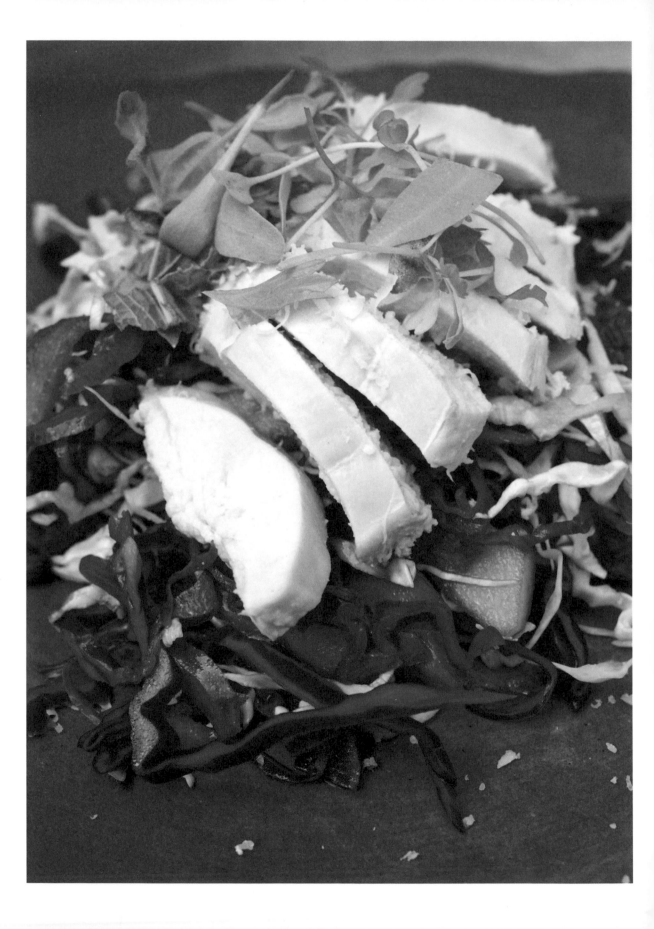

MATT MORAN
POACHED CHICKEN & CABBAGE SALAD

PREPARATION

1) Start by thinly slicing the red cabbage, then place in a bowl. Season cabbage with a tablespoon of salt. Cover and leave to one side for an hour. Then, using a sieve, rinse the cabbage under cold water and drain well.

2) Place the chardonnay vinegar in a pot and bring to the boil. Pour over the red cabbage and steep for an hour (alternatively, this could be done the day prior).

3) Place the chicken breast in a pot of seasoned water over a low heat and cook for 15 minutes with the lid on. Then remove the lid and allow to cool in the liquid.

4) Take the green cabbage and cut into thin slices. Place in a medium size bowl. Then cut the apple into thin batons and add to the bowl.

5) To make the vinaigrette, whisk together the vinegars, lemon juice, and mustard in a bowl. Season with salt and pepper, whisking constantly. Slowly pour in the oil until combined.

6) Remove the red cabbage from the liquid and drain, then add to the green cabbage and toss together lightly with the vinaigrette and season to taste.

7) Remove the chicken breast from the liquid and slice into thin strips.

8) To Serve: Divide the cabbage salad between 4 plates and arrange the strips of chicken breast on top. Shave over some parmesan and finish with some baby shiso leaves to garnish.

INGREDIENTS

(Serves 4)

» ¼ red cabbage
» ⅞ cup / 200 ml chardonnay vinegar
» ¼ green cabbage
» 1 large chicken breast
» 1 green apple
» 1 tbsp white wine vinegar
» 1 tbsp champagne vinegar
» 1 tbsp lemon juice
» 1 tbsp Dijon mustard
» ⅖ cup / 80 ml grape seed oil
» Salt and pepper

Garnish:
» Parmesan
» ½ package baby shiso leaves

MATT MORAN

Matt Moran is an Australian celebrity chef known for being a guest on various TV cooking shows in Asia, Europe, and Australia. Matt has many successful and iconic restaurants in Australia including Aria, Chiswick, and North Bondi Fish. He has written multiple cookbooks and is also a member of the international culinary panel for Singapore Airlines.

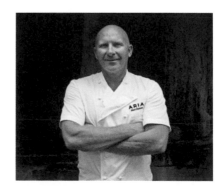

THE PLANT CAFÉ
SAUTÉED VEGETABLES OVER QUINOA WITH FRESH HERB & MISO-GINGER SAUCE

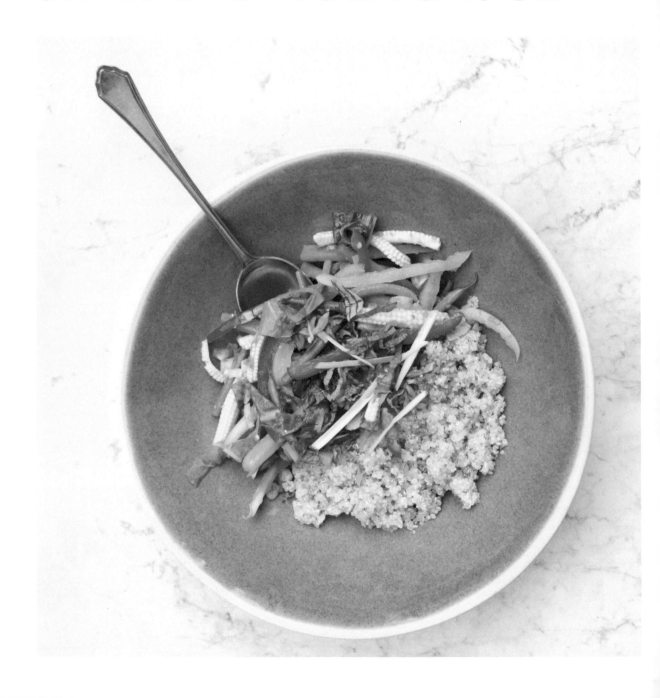

PREPARATION

Miso-Ginger sauce:
1) Heat the oil in a sauté pan over medium-high heat;
   add the onion and sauté until caramelized.
2) Combine the rest of the ingredients in a blender with
   the caramelized onions and purée until smooth. Set aside.

Quinoa:
1) Combine the quinoa, vegetable stock, and salt in
   a medium-size saucepan with a tight-fitting lid.
2) Place the pan over high heat with the lid on and cook
   until steam starts to escape; turn the heat down low and
   allow the quinoa to cook for 20 minutes.
3) Turn off the heat and let the quinoa sit for 5 minutes,
   then remove the lid and fluff quinoa with a fork.
4) Add additional salt to taste.

Vegetable Sauté:
1) Heat a large sauté pan over high heat.
2) Add the oil, then the garlic. Cook for about 30 seconds,
   until the garlic is fragrant.
3) Add the vegetables, cook until soft, then add ¾ cup / 180 ml
   of the miso-ginger sauce or more to taste. Add optional
   ingredients at this time and continue to cook until the sauce
   has coated the vegetables.

To Serve:
1) Divide the cooked quinoa into 6 bowls, top with
   the vegetable sauté and chopped herbs.

THE PLANT CAFÉ

With a mission to promote the well-being of people and the planet,
The Plant Café grew out of a desire to make it easy and affordable
to eat delicious healthy, local food. The San Francisco-based café
serves dishes made with 100% organic and local ingredients.
The menu is a diverse composition of contemporary California
cuisine with Asian-inspired flavors.

INGREDIENTS

(Serves 6)

Miso-Ginger Sauce:
» 2 tsp neutral-flavored oil
» ½ cup / 75 g red onion
  (peeled and diced)
» ¼ cup / 60 g white miso
» ¼ cup / 60 g red miso
» 1 tbsp agave nectar
» ½ cup / 120 ml vegetable stock
  or water
» 2 tbsp toasted sesame oil
» ¼ cup / 60 ml lemon juice
» ¼ cup / 15 g ginger
  (peeled and chopped)
» 1 tbsp tamari soy sauce

Quinoa:
» 2 cups / 340 g quinoa,
  (rinsed and drained in a strainer)
» 3 cups / 720 ml vegetable stock
  or water
» Sea salt to taste

Vegetable Sauté:
» 1 tbsp neutral-flavored oil
» 1 tbsp garlic (minced)
» 8 cups / 560–700 g mixed vegetables (e.g. broccoli, carrots, corn,
  bok choy, carrots, bell peppers)
  (peeled and cut into bite size pieces)
» 1 cup / 140 g grilled chicken breast
  (shredded), baked tofu (cubed),
  or shrimp (cooked, peeled,
  deveined) (optional)

Garnish:
» 3 tbsp mixed herbs (chopped)
  (e.g. basil, mint, and cilantro)

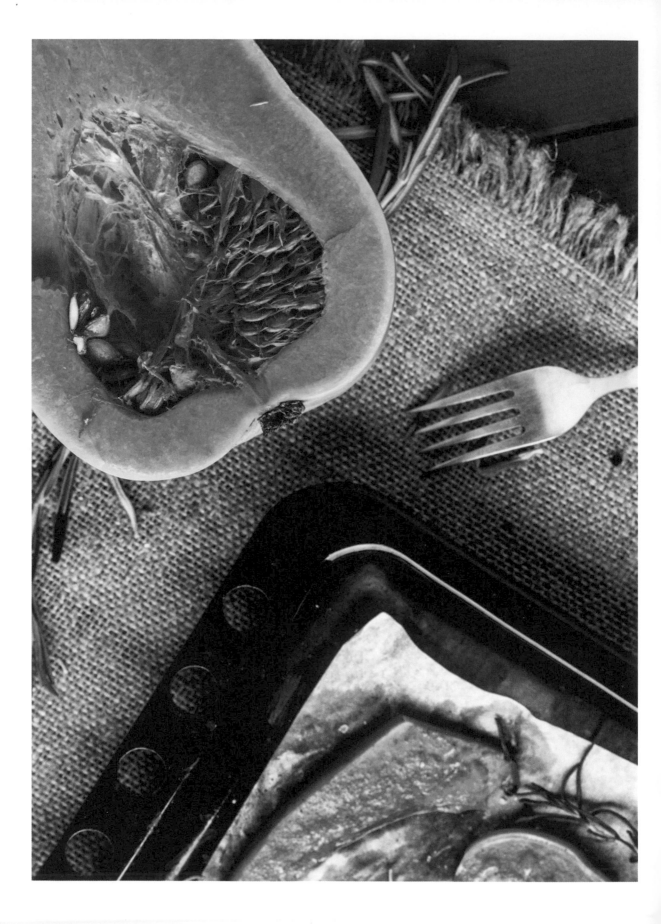

STEPH ADAMS

ROAST PUMPKIN WITH GOAT CHEESE

PREPARATION

1) Preheat the oven to 350°F / 180°C.

2) Cut the pumpkin into cubes and place into a roasting pan.

3) Sauté with olive oil, garlic, salt, and pepper.

4) Roast in oven for 30–40 minutes.

5) Place the pumpkin into a serving bowl and garnish with avocado, basil, and goat cheese.

INGREDIENTS

» *½ pumpkin*
» *2 tsp olive oil*
» *2–3 garlic cloves*
» *½ avocado*
» *5 basil leaves*
» *½ packet soft goat cheese*
» *Salt and pepper to taste*

STEPH SAYS:

"So nutritious and quick to make!"

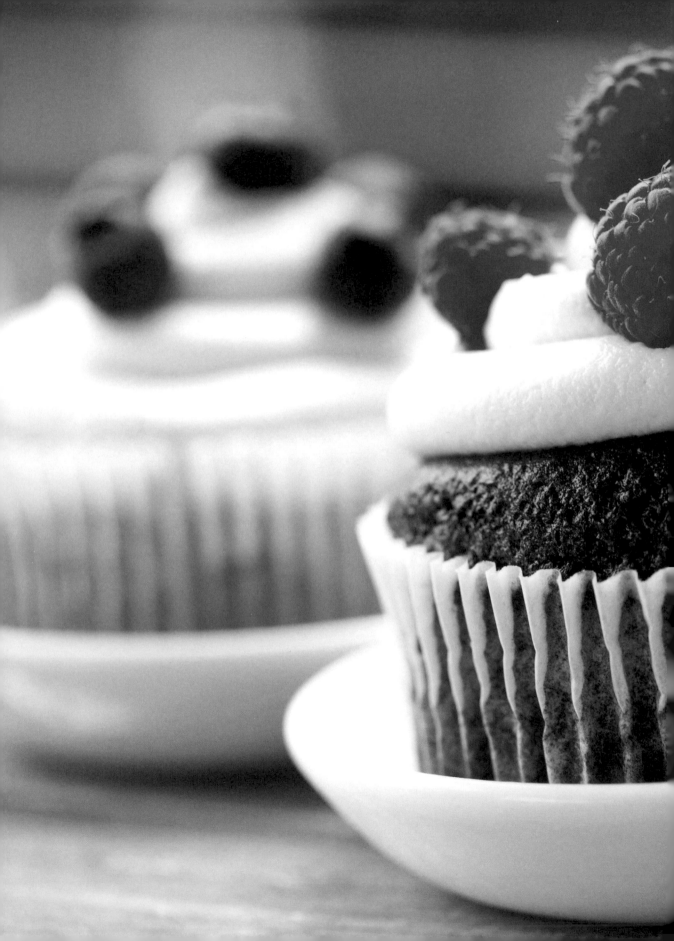

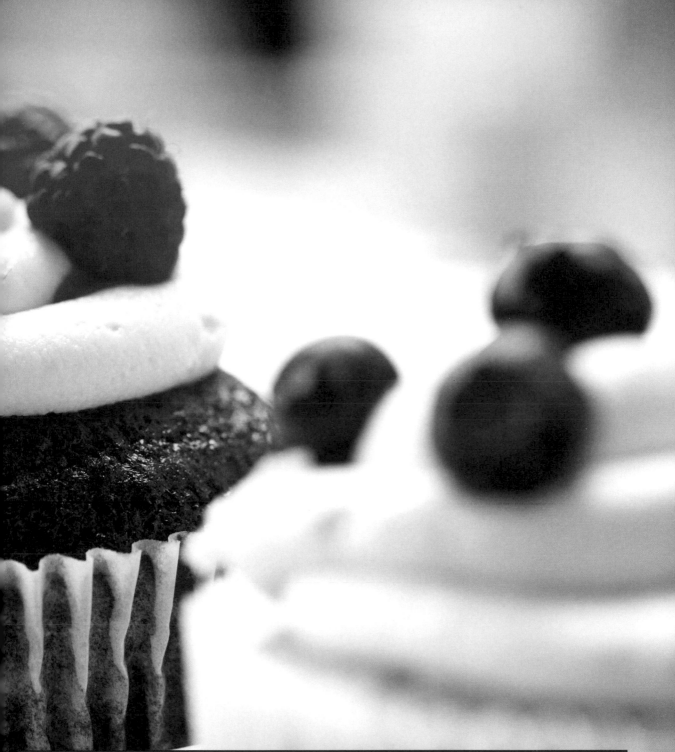

CHAPTER 4

SNACKS & SWEETS

I WANT CANDY

Who said that healthy food can't be delicious? These dishes are perfect desserts or treats on their own for people with a sweet tooth who also want to nourish their bodies with clean, wholesome ingredients. Kids and big kids alike will all enjoy these delightful and healthy indulgences.

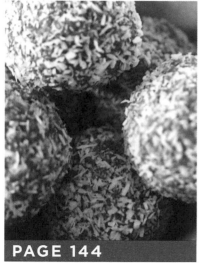

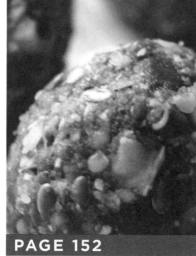

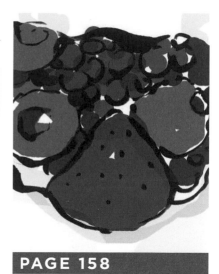

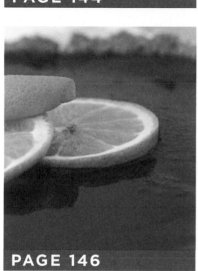

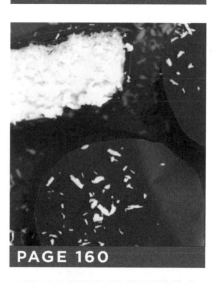

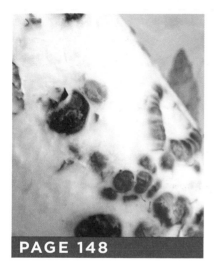

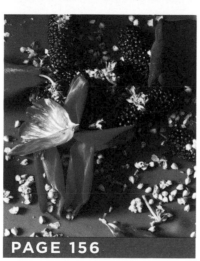

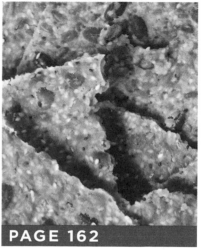

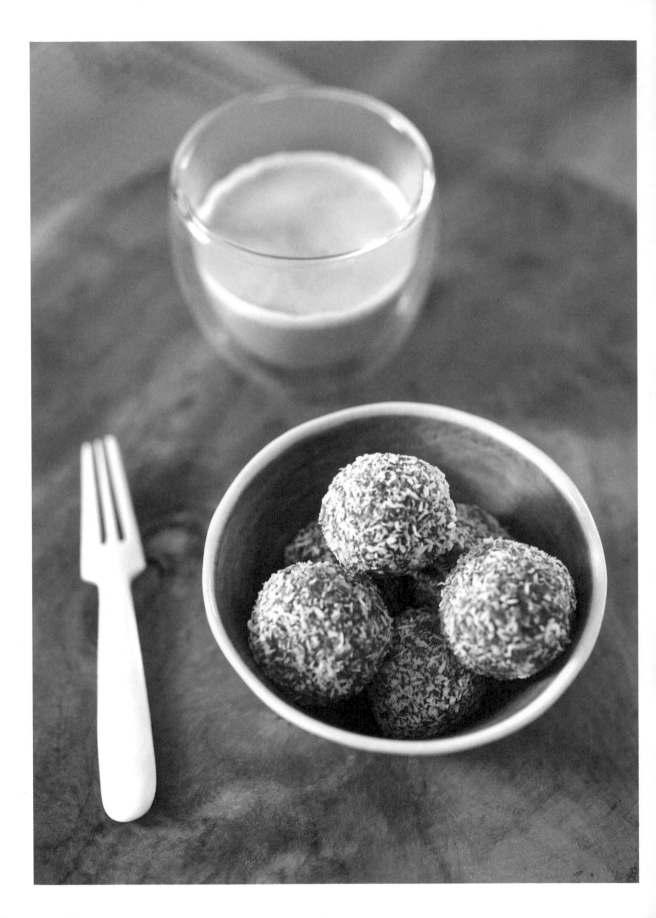

MELISSA ODABASH
FITNESS BALLS

PREPARATION

1) In a food processor, blend almonds, cacao powder, chia seeds, and protein powder together, then transfer into a bowl.

2) Blend the dates until they form a paste.

3) Slowly add the bowl of blended almonds into the food processor together with the coconut oil.

4) If you need to add more liquid, carefully add a little water to help the mixture stick together.

5) Roll the paste into 1-in. / 2.5 cm balls, then roll in the desiccated coconut.

6) Put them in the fridge to harden.

INGREDIENTS

» *10 Medjool dates (pitted)*
» *2 cups / 280 g almonds*
» *2 scoops of vanilla protein powder*
» *1 tbsp chia seeds*
» *2 tbsp raw cacao powder*
» *1 tbsp coconut oil*
» *Desiccated coconut*

MELISSA ODABASH

Former swimsuit model, Melissa Odabash, lived and worked in Italy for many years before she launched her swimwear collection in 1999. Her collection swiftly came to epitomize the glamour and sophistication of a luxury lifestyle brand, and British *Vogue* was quick to name it "The Ferraris of the bikini world." In 2014, Melissa was honored with the title "Designer of the year" at the Mode City Fashion Show in Paris. Melissa's collections are distributed in more than 50 countries and throughout 300 luxury department stores, boutiques, and resorts. With her continuing global success, Melissa has teamed up with many high-profile stars and brands, creating new outlets for her ever-growing following.

www.odabash.com

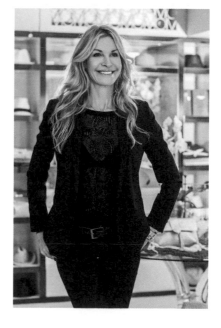

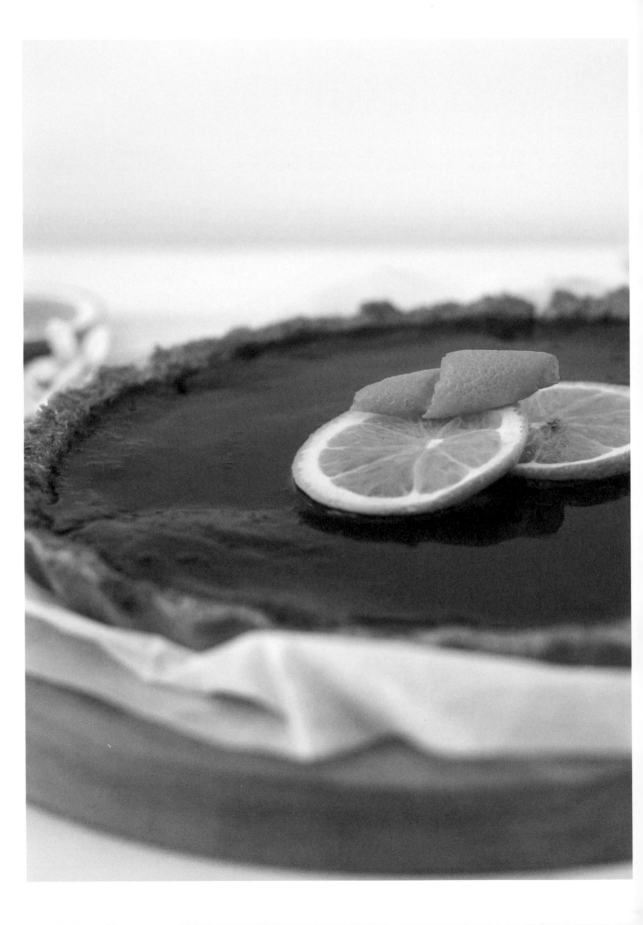

MELISSA AMBROSINI
CHOCOLATE & ORANGE TART

PREPARATION

Base:
1) Blend all base ingredients in food processor.
2) Line the base of a pie pan with non-stick paper. Press base mixture into the pan and up the sides about ½-in. / 1 cm high. Make it packed down and firm.
3) Bake in an oven on 280°F / 140°C degrees until golden brown, then remove from oven to cool.

Filling:
1) To make the filling, whisk eggs in a saucepan. Add coconut oil and place on a gentle heat until oil is melted into eggs. Sir constantly to avoid the eggs clumping.
2) Once melted, add orange juice, orange zest, cacao, and stevia. Keep stirring until the mixture starts to get silky. Avoid it getting too thick as the oil will separate.
3) Take off heat. Press the mixture through a strainer into the cooled base, leaving only the zest in the strainer. (Be sure to scrape the filling off the bottom of the strainer!)
4) Shake the pan until filling covers the whole base evenly.
5) Place in fridge to set (approximately 2 hours).
6) Serve with grated orange zest (or orange slices) on top.

INGREDIENTS

Base:
» 2 ½ cups / 220 g desiccated coconut
» ½ tsp vanilla bean powder
» ½ tsp ground cinnamon
» 4 tbsp coconut oil
» 1 egg
» Pinch of salt
» ½ tsp liquid stevia

Filling:
» Juice and zest of 2 oranges
» ¼ tsp liquid stevia (or to taste)
» 3 eggs
» 6 tbsp coconut oil
» 3 tbsp cacao powder
» 2 tbsp cacao butter (melted)

MELISSA AMBROSINI

Melissa Ambrosini is an author, speaker, lifestyle entrepreneur, and self-love teacher. Melissa's mission is to inspire women to master their inner "Mean Girl" and to become wildly wealthy, fabulously healthy, and bursting with love.

www.melissaambrosini.com

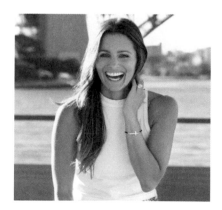

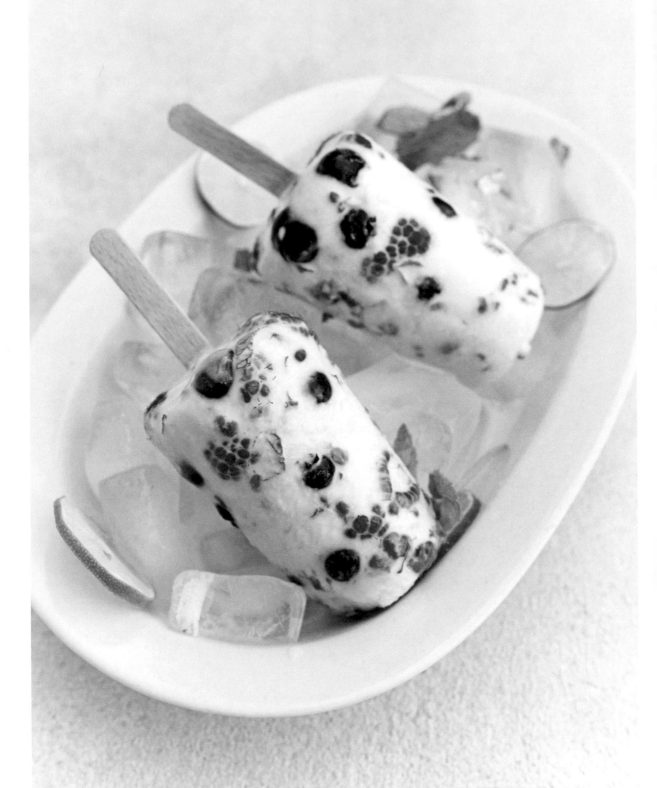

TALI SHINE
COCOBERRY ICICLES

PREPARATION

1) Mix the coconut cream and rice malt syrup in a bowl.

2) Stir berries and coconut cream mixture together.

3) Scatter a few mint leaves into the mixture.

4) Pour the mixture into ice cube molds.

5) Place a popsicle stick in each mold.

6) Place in freezer and serve once cubes are frozen.

INGREDIENTS

» 1 ¼ cups / 300 ml coconut cream
» ¼ cup / 50 g strawberries (chopped)
» ½ cup / 50 g raspberries
» ⅖ cup / 50 g blueberries
» 1 tsp rice malt syrup
» 1 small bunch of mint
» 6 popsicle sticks

TALI SAYS:

"These cocoberry icicles are the perfect hot summer's treat. I love eating them on warm afternoons, as well as serving them for dessert at dinner parties. It brings out the childhood joy in all."

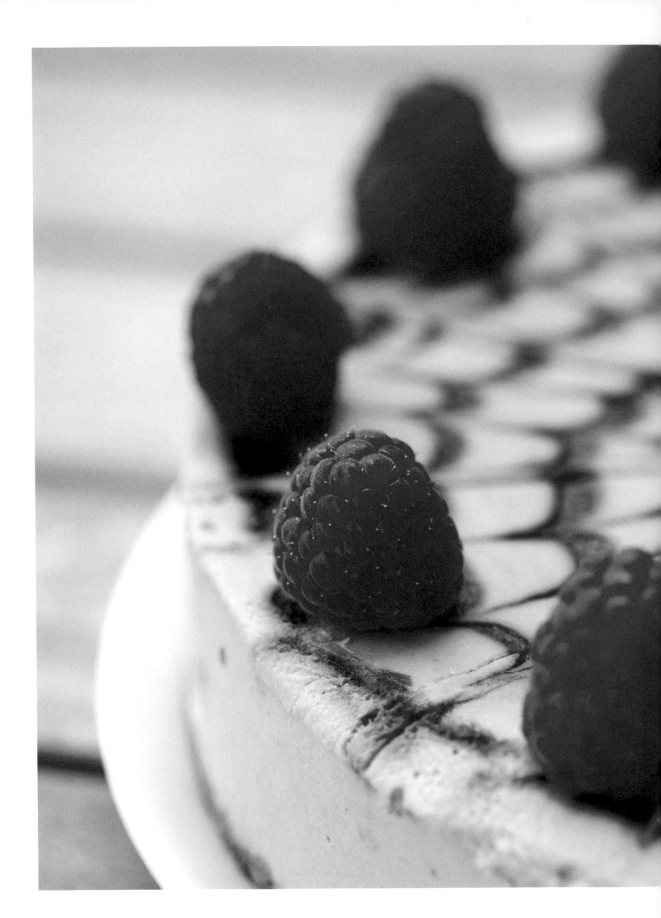

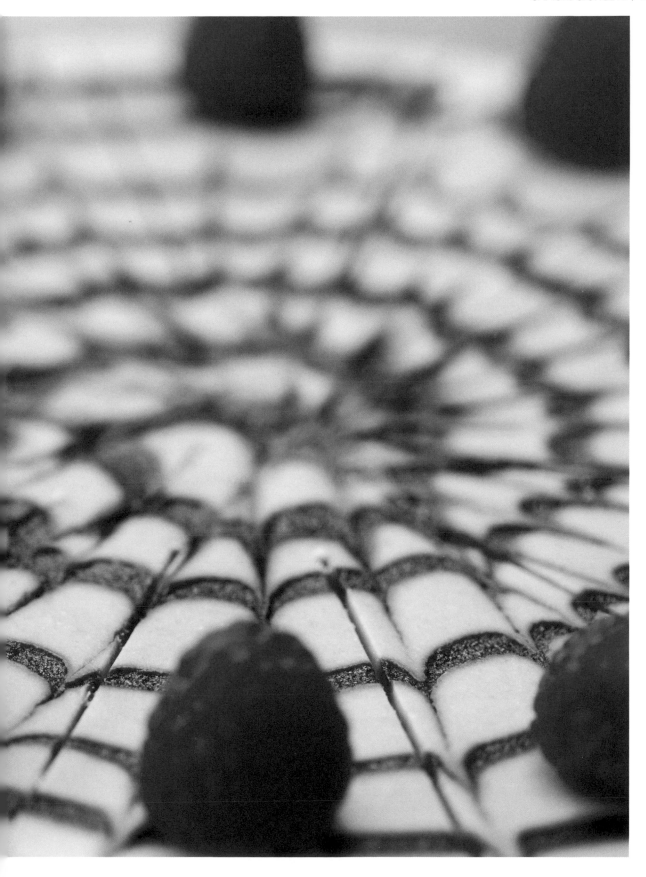

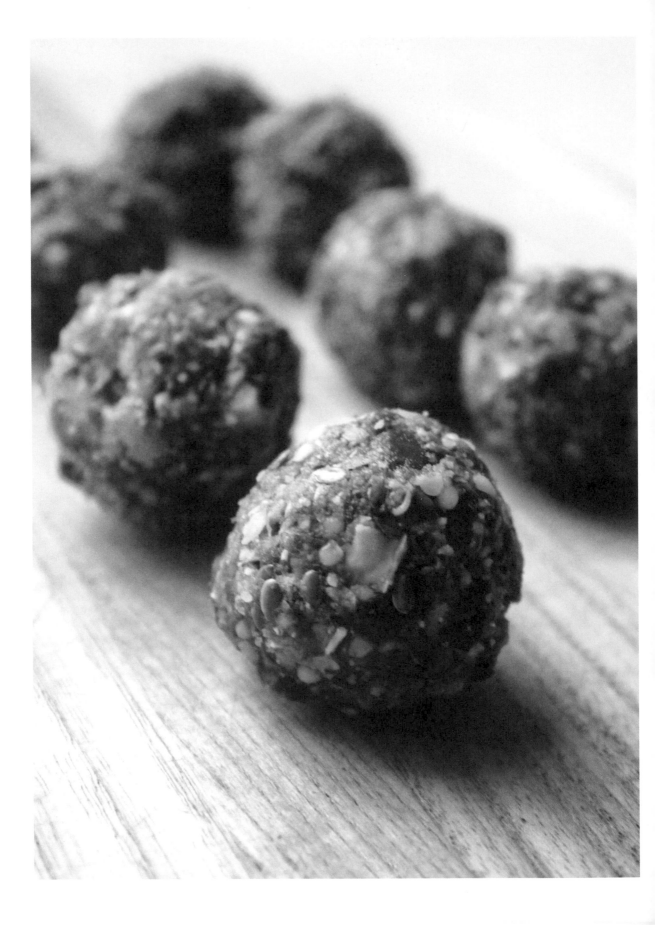

MY GOODNESS
MATCHA ENERGY BALLS

PREPARATION

1) Place all of the dry ingredients into a blender, then mix together. While this is happening you can soak the dates in boiling water to soften them up. Once the dry ingredients are blended together in a fine powder, pour the powder into a bowl and set aside.

2) Next, place the dates into the blender and mix until they are mashed up. Add in part of the powder and continue blending. Once the first half is all blended, add the rest of the powder and give it a really good stir together with a spoon. It should all start to clump together.

3) Spoon out little lumps of the mixture and roll them into balls. Put them in the fridge to set before enjoying.

Good to Know:
For those who have never heard of this green super powder, matcha is a Japanese green tea packed full of antioxidants, vitamins, and minerals. It can also increase your concentration and performance. Mixed with seeds, dates, and nuts, this little power ball will keep you living life to the fullest! This recipe is super simple and will keep in the fridge for up to seven days, perfect for those big weeks.

INGREDIENTS

(Makes 10–12 balls)

- » ½ cup / 70 g pistachios
- » ½ cup / 70 g almonds
- » 2 tbsp flaxseeds
- » 2 tbsp hemp seeds
- » 1 ⅛ cups / 200 g pitted dates
- » 1 heaping tsp matcha powder
- » 1 tbsp maple syrup (if you prefer a little sweetener)

MY GOODNESS

Originally from the south coast of England, Izzy Reuss has lived in Berlin for two years with her German husband. After making the transition to a totally plant-based diet, free from refined sugars, preservatives, and chemicals, Izzy started to feel the health benefits in her everyday life. She had more energy, her skin started to glow, and because she felt better overall, that health started to flow into all areas of her life. In 2015, she founded My Goodness, a website and shop all about empowering people to live to their full potential by developing all-round healthy lifestyles.

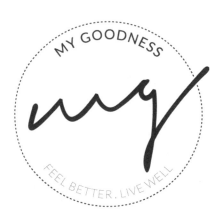

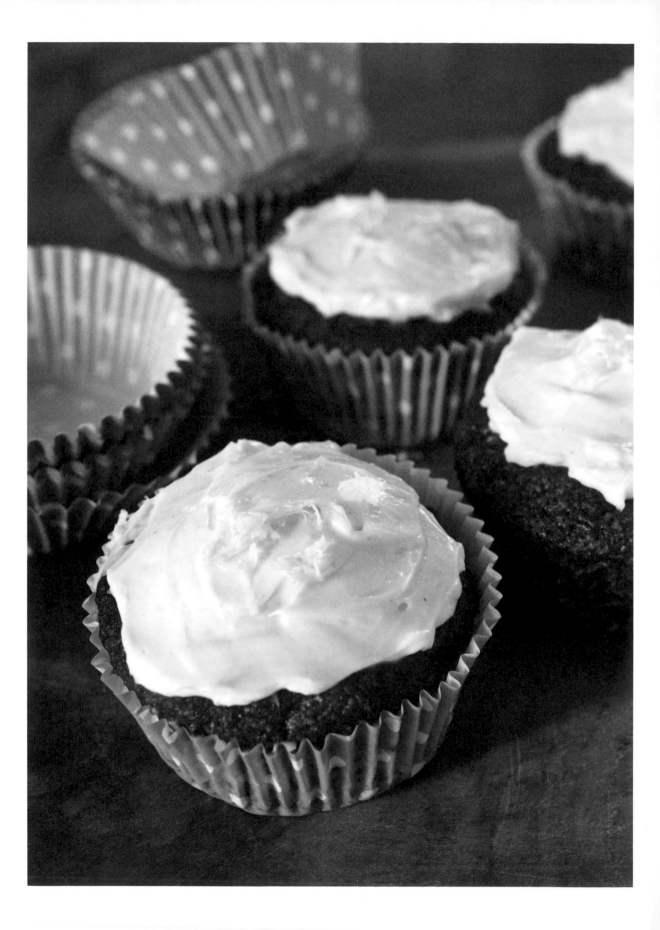

LOHRALEE ASTOR
SUGAR-FREE CARROT CUPCAKES

PREPARATION

1) Preheat the oven to 350°F / 180°C.

2) Sift the flour, baking soda, baking powder, salt, nutmeg, and cinnamon into a bowl.

3) In another bowl, mix together the milk, eggs, vanilla extract, oil, and xylitol. Slowly add in the dry ingredients and mix well.

4) Combine the carrots, lemon zest, desiccated coconut, and peaches in another bowl, then slowly add to the mixture.

5) Pour the mixture into a cupcake tin and bake for 10–15 minutes or until golden brown.

6) Once the cupcakes are in the oven, start the frosting. Combine the cream cheese, zest of lemon, and agave nectar and mix well.

7) When the cupcakes are cooked and cooled, apply frosting.

INGREDIENTS

(For 12 Cupcakes)
- » *1 cup / 120 g buckwheat flour*
- » *1 tsp baking soda*
- » *½ tsp baking powder*
- » *2 tsp cinnamon*
- » *1 tsp nutmeg*
- » *Pinch of sea salt*
- » *2 eggs*
- » *⅖ cup / 100 ml milk of your choice (rice, goat, cow, almond)*
- » *⅖ cup / 100 ml rapeseed oil*
- » *1 cup / 215 g xylitol*
- » *2 tsp vanilla extract*
- » *1 cup / 50 g grated carrots*
- » *1 cup / 90 g desiccated coconut*
- » *1 cup / 225 g finely chopped peaches in their natural juice*
- » *Zest of 1 lemon*

Zest of Lemon Frosting:
- » *1 ½ cups / 340 g cream cheese*
- » *3 tbsp agave nectar*
- » *Zest of 1 lemon*

LOHRALEE ASTOR

Former model Lohralee Astor is a sought-after London-based nutritional therapist. A member of the prestigious American/ European aristocratic Astor family, she loves entertaining both in London and in the English countryside and is always coming up with delicious, healthy dishes for her husband, children, extended family, and high-profile clientele.

www.lohra.co.uk

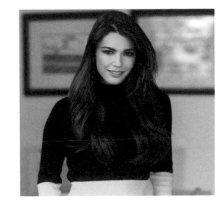

SALTED CHOC CARDAMOM GANACHE

SARAH WILSON

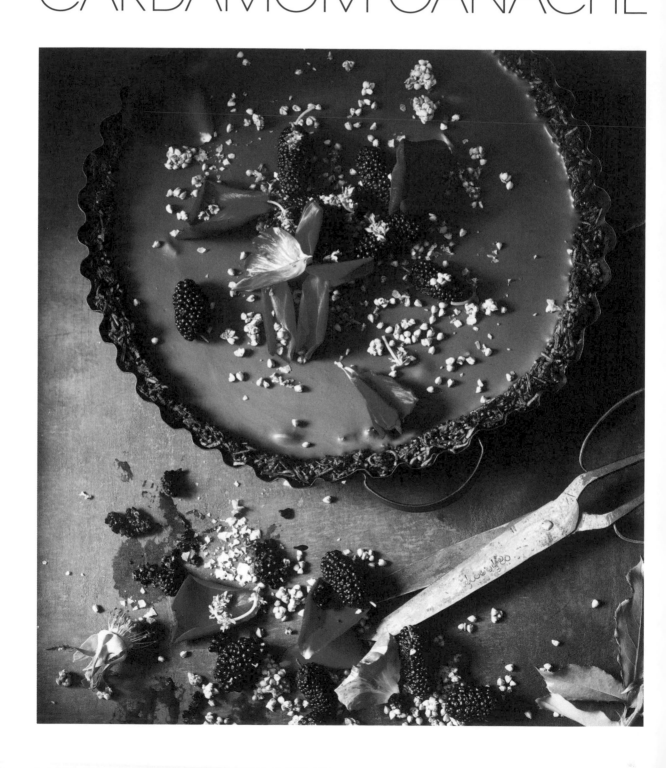

PREPARATION

1) Preheat the oven to 350°F / 180°C.
2) To make the crust, melt the coconut oil and rice malt syrup in a saucepan.
3) Remove saucepan from heat and add the shredded coconut and cacao powder, mix well.
4) Press the mixture into the base and up the side of a quiche or tart tin—no need to grease it—so that the mixture's approximately 0.2-in. / 5 mm thick all over.
5) Bake the crust for 15–20 minutes. Remove from the oven and set aside to cool and firm.
6) While the crust is cooling, heat the coconut cream, cardamom pods, and vanilla in a saucepan to a simmer, then turn off the heat and cover with a lid.
7) Allow filling mixture to steep for 10 minutes.
8) Strain the coconut cream mixture into a bowl, reserving ¼ cup in the pan for emergency use later, if needed. Discard the cardamom pods (or save to spice up chai tea).
9) Add the chocolate and salt into a bowl, whisking through until silky and melted.
10) If the fats separate and your ganache develops a chocolaty, cottage cheese appearance, just add the reserved coconut cream, whisking swiftly to bring it all back together.
11) Once silky, pour into the tart shell and refrigerate until the ganache sets (at least 2 hours).
12) Garnish with a pinch of coarse sea salt and berries, petals, and activated groaties, as desired.

INGREDIENTS

Crust:
» ⅓ cup / 70 g coconut oil
» ¼ cup / 90 g rice malt syrup
» 2 cups / 120 g shredded coconut
» 1 tbsp raw cacao powder

Filling:
» 1 scant cup / 270 ml canned coconut cream
» 2 tablespoons cardamom pods (lightly crushed with a flat blade until the outer husks crack)
» ½ tsp pure vanilla powder or 1 tsp pure vanilla extract
» 3.5 oz / 100 g dark chocolate (85–90% cocoa) (chopped)
» Pinch of sea salt, plus coarse sea salt
» Berries, edible flower petals, and activated groaties to garnish (optional)

SARAH WILSON

Sarah Wilson is a New York Times best-selling author and entrepreneur. Her career as a former journalist spanned 20 years across television, radio, magazines, newspapers, and online outlets. She's been the editor of *Cosmopolitan* magazine, hosted the first season of *MasterChef Australia*, and penned international best sellers including *I Quit Sugar*, *I Quit Sugar For Life* and *I Quit Sugar: Simplicious*. Outside of her professional life, Sarah bikes everywhere and loves to hike.

www.sarahwilson.com

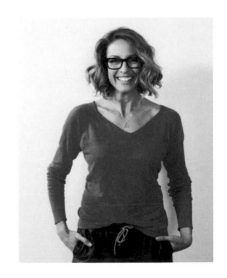

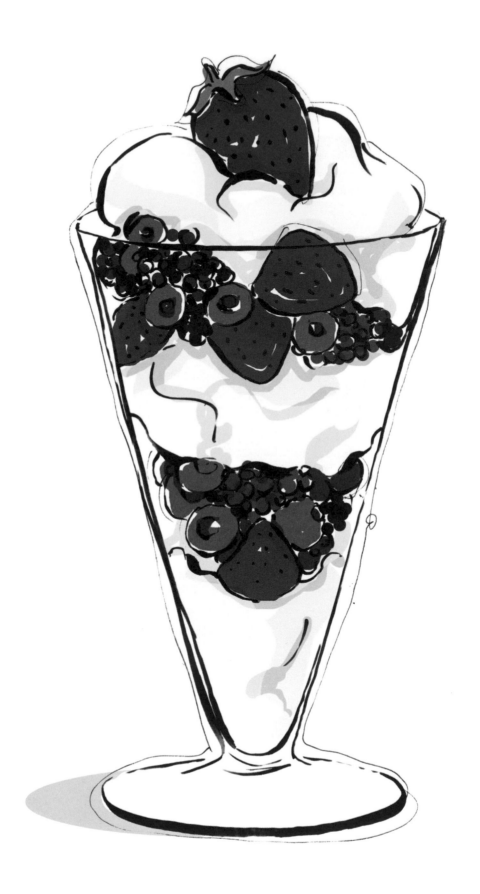

MEGAN HESS
YOGURT BERRY SWIRL

PREPARATION

1) Wash and remove storks from strawberries and slice into quarters.

2) Swirl strawberries and mixed berries through yogurt and serve.

INGREDIENTS

» *1 heaping cup / 200 g fresh or frozen berries*
» *1 package fresh strawberries*
» *1 cup / 250 g Greek yogurt (or sheep or coconut yogurt)*

MEGAN HESS

Megan Hess is an international fashion illustrator who works with some of the most prestigious fashion designers and luxury brands around the world such as Chanel, Dior, Cartier, Montblanc, and Tiffany & Co.

www.meganhess.com

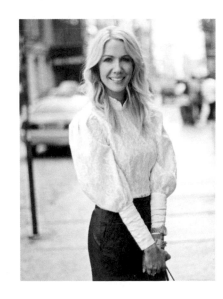

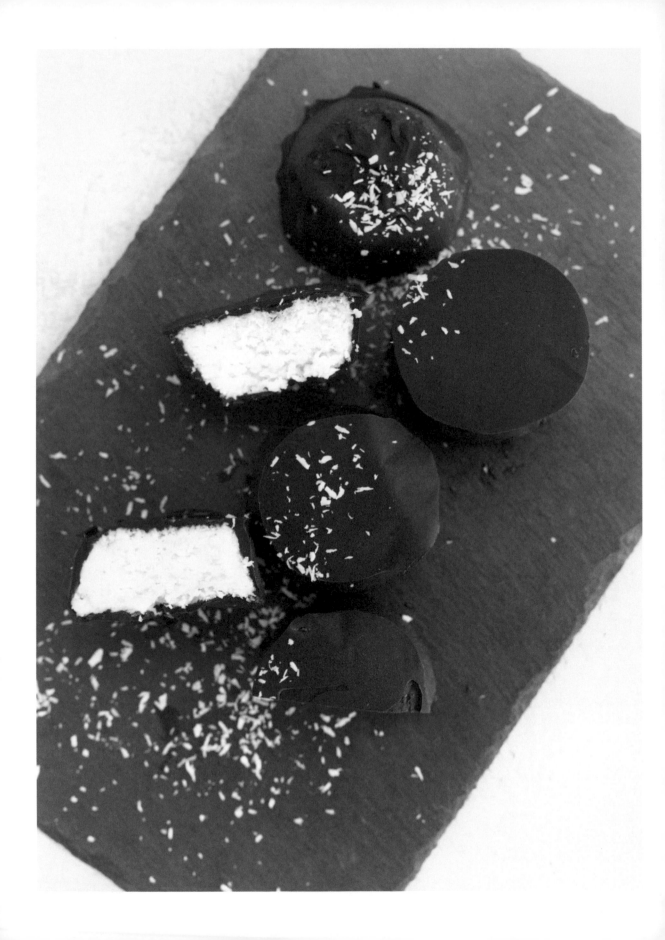

TALI SHINE
VEGAN RAW CHOC COCO BITES

PREPARATION

1) Add shredded coconut, coconut cream, coconut milk, and maple syrup into a blender and pulse to create a thick mixture.
2) Grease a baking tray with coconut oil.
3) Making sure that your hands are clean, then make rectangles or cylinders of the mixture. You can also press the mixture into a mini muffin pan or ice cube tray to form more consistent shapes.
4) Place the baking tray in the fridge or freezer to allow mixture to set.
5) To make the coating, add coconut oil, cacao powder, and maple syrup into a small pot.
6) On a low heat, stir mixture until it is combined.
7) Set aside to cool.
8) Remove the coconut mixture from the fridge or freezer.
9) Using chopsticks or two spoons, dip one piece in the raw chocolate mixture, making sure that all sides are covered.
10) Place chocolate-covered pieces back into the fridge or freezer to set.
11) Once the raw chocolate has set, take them out and repeat the dipping process to allow a thicker covering.
12) Place in an air-tight container and store in the fridge.

INGREDIENTS

Filling:
» *1 ½ cups / 120 g raw shredded coconut*
» *¼ cup / 60 g coconut milk*
» *¼ cup / 75 g coconut cream*
» *2 tbsp maple syrup*

Raw Chocolate Coating:
» *¼ cup / 55 g coconut oil*
» *¼ cup / 30 g raw cacao powder*
» *1 tbsp maple syrup*

TALI SAYS:

"When you don't want the kids to have all of the fun, enjoy this delicious treat. Coconut is not only filled with protein, but also good fats that will keep your hair, skin, and nails in great condition."

GLUTEN-FREE SEED CRACKERS

GRETHA SCHOLTZ

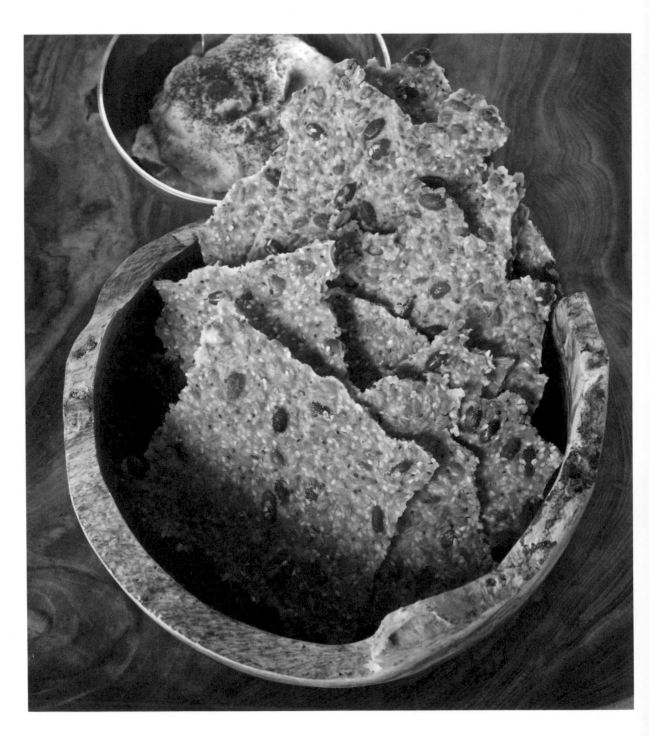

PREPARATION

1) Preheat oven to 300°F / 150°C with the shelf on the middle oven rack.

2) Cut 2 pieces of baking paper the size of a baking tray.

3) Mix all dry ingredients together in a bowl.

4) Add the oil and boiling water into the bowl and mix together until it turns into a smooth mass of cracker dough.

5) Put some of the dough onto one piece of baking paper and flatten slightly with the palm of your hand.

6) Put the other sheet of baking paper on top and roll as thinly as possible with a rolling pin, trying to get the mass the same size as the baking paper.

7) Cut off the excess bits of cracker dough and put it back in the bowl to be rolled out on the next baking tray.

8) Slide the rolled out dough onto the baking sheet and remove the top piece of baking paper.

9) If you want the crackers more salty, sprinkle some sea salt on top and lightly press it into the dough with the back of your hand.

10) Keep the leftover dough in the bowl with a piece of cling-film over it until you have a free baking sheet and space in the oven to bake the next batch. If the dough gets too dry, just add a few drops of hot water before rolling it out.

11) Bake for about 1 hour. The crackers should be nice and crisp by then. Remove and let cool.

12) Break the crackers into any size you like.

13) Store in an air-tight container. The crackers can be put in a sealable plastic bag and freeze very well. No need to defrost before eating.

INGREDIENTS

» 1 cup / 120 g yellow corn flour
» 1 cup / 140 g potato starch or cornstarch
» ½ cup / 80 g golden flaxseeds (normal flaxseeds will also work)
» ½ cup / 75 g sesame seeds
» ½ cup / 100 g pumpkin seeds
» ¾ cup / 110 g sunflower seeds
» 2 tbsp chia seeds
» 1 tsp fine table salt or Himalayan pink salt
» ¼ cup / 60 ml extra-virgin olive oil
» ¼ cup / 50 ml sunflower or canola oil
» 1 cup / 240 ml boiling water

Note: If you can't find yellow corn flour, you can use 1 cup / 140 g of potato starch and 1 cup / 140 g of cornstarch, or 2 cups / 280 g of cornstarch only.

The seed mix is not set in stone. Just use what you like and what you have on hand, in total about 2 ¼ cups / 340 g of seeds.

GRETHA SCHOLTZ

Food has always played a central role in Gretha Scholtz's life. She grew up on a farm in Africa before traveling the world in her teens and twenties as a model, exposing her to food from all corners of the globe. Discovering exciting new flavors ignited her passion for blending ingredients that transcend borders and traditions. Now an interior designer, Gretha spends her life traveling with her husband, Mogens Tholstrup, between South Africa, Finland, France, and Switzerland.

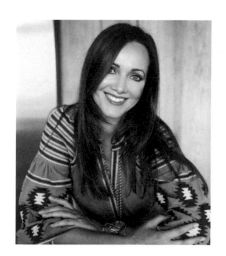

INDEX

We believe in buying seasonal and organic produce. If you are not in a position to buy organic then we recommend making sure that your proteins such as meat, poultry, and eggs are organic and your fish is wild-caught.

SERVICES

ARCADE CAFÉ (P. 96)
152 Bree Street (corner Pepper Street)
Cape Town
South Africa
http://arcadecafe.co.za

BODYISM LONDON (PP. 108, 126)
222 – 224 Westbourne Grove
London W11 2RH
United Kingdom
www.bodyism.com
www.cleanandlean.com

CAFÉ GRATITUDE (P. 84)
639 N. Larchmont Blvd
Los Angeles, CA
USA
Phone: +1 323 5806 383
http://cafegratitude.com

CAPRI PALACE HOTEL & SPA (P. 90)
Via Capodimonte 14
80071 Anacapri (NA), Capri
Italy
Phone: +39 08 19780 111
www.capripalace.com

COMO SHAMBALA ESTATE (P. 58)
Banjar Begawan, Desa Melinggih Kelod
Payangan. Ubud, Gianyar
Bali 80571
Indonesia
Phone: +62 361 978 888
www.comohotels.com/comoshambhalaestate

CRUDE JUICE (P. 36)
www.crudejuice.co.uk

DALUMA (P. 100)
Weinbergsweg 3
10119 Berlin
Germany
Phone: +49 30 2095 0255
www.daluma.de

DE KAS (P. 46)
Kamerlingh Onneslaan 3
1097 DE Amsterdam
Netherlands
Phone: +31 20 462 45 62
www.restaurantdekas.nl

GLOW HEALTHBAR (P. 118)
Viktoriastrasse 3
3780 Gstaad
Switzerland
Phone: + 41 26 674 60 10
http://glowhealthbar.ch

GRACE BELGRAVIA (P. 114)
11c West Halkin Street
London SW1X 8JL
United Kingdom
Phone: +44 20 7235 8900
www.gracebelgravia.com

HARRY'S BONDI (P. 74)
2/136 Wairoa Avenue,
Bondi Beach NSW 2026
Australia
Phone: +61 2 9130 2180
http://harrysbondi.com.au

HOTEL ARTS BARCELONA (P. 132)
Marina 19–21
08005 Barcelona
Spain
Phone: +34 93 221 10 00
www.hotelartsbarcelona.com

IMBIBERY LONDON (P. 34)
www.imbiberylondon.com

LAURA'S DELI (P. 50)
Carlsplatz 1
40213 Düsseldorf
Germany
Phone: +49 211 8693 3880
www.laurasdeli.de

MILTON PARK COUNTRY HOUSE
HOTEL & SPA (P. 130)
Horderns Road, Bowral NSW 2576
Australia
Phone: +61 2 4861 8100
www.miltonpark.com.au

MY GOODNESS (P. 152)
www.mygoodnessberlin.com

THE PLANT CAFÉ (P. 136)
Suite 108, Pier 3, The Embarcadero
San Francisco, CA 94111
USA
Phone: +1 415 9840 437
www.theplantcafe.com

PLENISH CLEANSE (P. 24)
www.plenishcleanse.com

POINT YAMU BY COMO (P. 86)
225 Moo 7
Pa Klok, Talang, Phuket 83110
Thailand
Phone: +66 7 636 0100
www.comohotels.com/pointyamu

PORCH AND PARLOUR (P. 60)
17-18/110 Ramsgate Ave,
North Bondi NSW 2026
Australia
Phone: +61 2 9300 0111
www.porchandparlour.com

RAE'S ON WATEGOS (P. 124)
6 – 8 Marine Parade
Byron Bay NSW 2481
Australia
Phone: +61 2 6685 5366
www.raes.com.au

SEXY FOOD (P. 92)
190 Bree Street
Cape Town
South Africa
Phone: +27 21 422 5445
www.sexyfood.co.za

SOUTH KENSINGTON CLUB (P. 32)
38-42 Harrington Road
London SW7 3ND
United Kingdom
Phone: +44 20 3006 6868
www.southkensingtonclub.com

THE STORE KITCHEN (P. 64)
Soho House Berlin
Torstraße 1
10119 Berlin
Germany
Phone: +49 30 4050 4455 0
www.thestores.com

TRIBE 112 CAFÉ (P. 54)
The Studios, 112 Buitengracht Street,
Cape Town City Centre,
Cape Town 8000
South Africa
Phone: +27 72 736 6142
www.tribecoffee.co.za

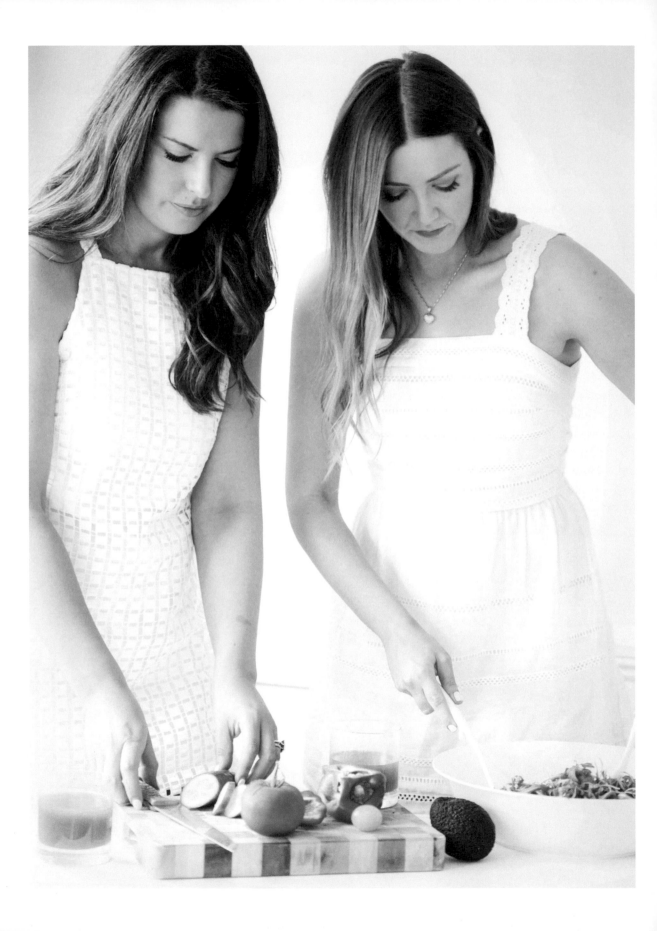

AUTHORS

Tali Shine

Tali is a health and wellness expert who consults for international spas and wellness centers, such as London's prestigious South Kensington Club, whose spa, fitness program, and juice bar she helped to develop. She also worked with clean-eating franchise Counter Kitchen to create healthy and delicious on-the-go dishes. With a Masters degree in journalism, Tali is often called upon by international television and print media to comment on wellness and lifestyle trends. She has written for numerous publications on the subjects of health, nutrition, beauty, and wellness. This has given her the opportunity to spend time with global experts and learn about important advancements in an array of lifestyle topics. A fan of travel, Tali is the author of *The Glam Girl's Guide to Sydney Shopping* and has worked with tourism boards. In 2005, she launched her own cosmetics line, Tali by Tali Shine, for the "girl on the go". The range is inspired by her favorite cities. Tali currently splits her time between London and Sydney.

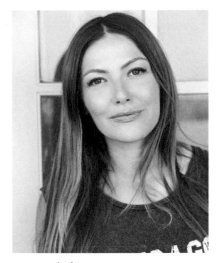

www.talishine.com
Instagram: @talishine

Steph Adams

Steph Adams is a digital influencer, former model, and art director. After eight years in the modeling industry flying around the world for commercial and magazine shoots, Steph started working as a designer for Australian *Vogue*, *GQ*, *Vogue Entertaining & Travel*, and *Vogue Living*. She then moved on to work as an art director for *Marie Claire* Australia and *Gourmet Traveller*, and other international publications including British *Vogue*, *Harper's Bazaar*, *Elle*, *Condé Nast Traveler*, and *Net-a-Porter* in London. Highly respected in the fashion industry, Steph continues to collaborate with brands and charities as a model, brand stylist, creative director, and ambassador. Steph's style and taste has been called upon to produce creative concepts for fashion's top brands like Chanel, Dior, Louis Vuitton, L'Oréal Paris, Tiffany & Co., Tag Heuer, SK-II, Shiseido, Skyy Vodka, and Max Factor.

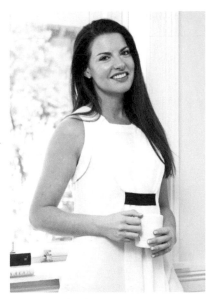

www.stephadams.com
Instagram: @stephadams2012

FOLLOW US ON INSTAGRAM

@talishine

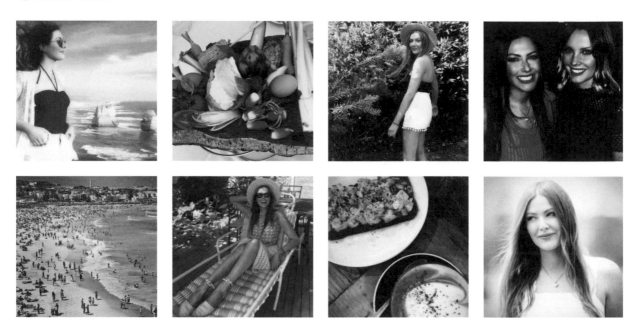

@stephadams2012

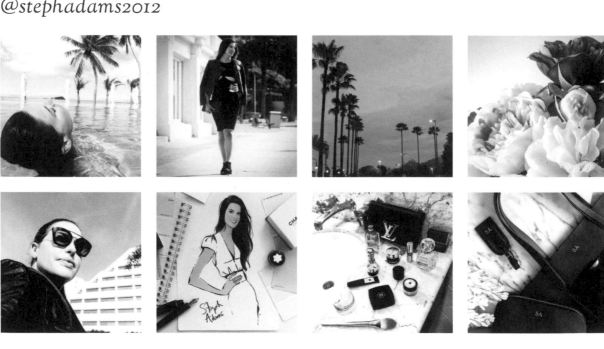

THANK YOUS & PHOTO CREDITS

Tali

Thank you to Siobhan, Jamie, Orla, and Niamh—the best people I know. Thank you for your unwavering support and love from all corners of the globe. Malin, Adriana, Sammy, Caroline, Julia, Sogol, Tijana, Rich, Lizzie, Celine, Katrina, Johanna, Alex, Joe, Nicky, and Bruce, Lynda, and Lauren, Ellie, Tim, Lynz, Denee, Tim, Lisa, BB, Mon, Mandy, Masha, Lee, Tigs and Skye. Steph and the amazing contributors, many of whom I am blessed to also call friends, particularly Danai, LL, Gabi, Deb, Matt, and Sarah. Thank you for making my dreams a reality, and for over a decade of friendship, Patrycia. Finally thank you for being there always, my rock, Papa Bear.

Steph

I would like to thank my mum and dad, my sister, Jules, and my husband, Joel, for your endless love and support. To the poeple who helped make this book a reality; Bianca, Nekes, Tali, Christiane and James, Rebecca, Lorna, Ash, Melissa, Megan, Sam, Elle, Andrea, Regina, Regine, and Patrycia. Without you all, this book may never have happened. I would also like to thank my very close friends: Sam Brett, and Jennifer Munroe, and last but not least, Annaliese who was diagnosed with breast cancer in the middle of working on this book. Your strength, bravery, and outlook on life is such an inspiration to me.

Cover front: © Nikki To (Harry's Bondi)
Cover back: © Patrycia Lukas Photography (top), © Chantell Bianchi (middle), © This is an extract from *I Quit Sugar: Simplicious* by Sarah Wilson, published by Pan Macmillan, RRP $39.99 (bottom left), © Mirjam Knickriem (bottom right)

All photos by Patrycia Lukas Photography except:
p. 1–2: © Chantell Bianchi, p. 11: (top) © iStock.com/Moncherie, (middle) © iStock.com/5PH, p. 12: © Courtesy of Daluma, Ailine Liefeld, p. 13: © Andreas Kuschner/Alimonie Design, p. 14: © Courtesy of My Goodness, p. 15: (bottom) © Courtesy of Daluma, Ailine Liefeld, p. 21: © WelleCo/Ben Blackall, p. 23 © iStock.com/eskymaks, p. 25: © Courtesy of Plenish Cleanse London, p. 26–27 © Eden Grill, p. 28–29: © Courtesy of Daluma, Ailine Liefeld, p. 31: © David Wheeler, p. 33: © Courtesy of South Kensington Club, p. 35: © Courtesy of Imbibery London, p. 37: © Courtesy of Crude Juice, p. 38: © Shutterstock.com/zi3000, p. 44: © Shutterstock.com/Vladislav Nosik, p. 47: © Ronald Hoeben, p. 50: © Courtesy of Laura's Deli, p. 51: © Andreas Kuschner/Alimonie Design, p. 53: © ModeSportif, p. 58–59: © Courtesy of COMO Hotels, p. 60: © Steph Adams, p. 61 and p. 63: © Luc Remond, p. 69: © Chantell Bianchi, p. 72: © Shutterstock.com/istetiana, p. 74–75: © Nikki To, p. 82: © Shutterstock.com/B. and E. Dudzinscy, p. 83: © Matt Benfell, p. 85: © Nicholas Roberts, p. 86-87: © Courtesy of COMO Hotels, p. 88: © Shutterstock.com/AnastasiaKopa, p. 89: © Attila Szilvasi, p. 90: © Courtesy of Capri Palace, p. 91: © eikona.eu, p. 100–101: © Courtesy of Daluma, Ailine Liefeld, p. 102: © Shutterstock.com/MShev, p. 103: © Bowen Arico, p. 105: © Courtesy of Lorna Jane, p. 106–107: © Mirjam Knickriem, p. 109: © Kate Davis-McLeod, p. 113: © Courtesy of Rachael Finch, p. 115: © Tom Sullam Photography, p. 118–121: © Raphael Fauy/Gstaadphotography.com, p. 121: © Nikolas Kominis/Studio Kominis, p. 123: © Courtesy of Gabriela Peacock, p. 124: © Sarah Gray, p. 125: © Courtesy of Rae's on Wategos, p. 126–127: © Kate Davis-McLeod, p. 129: © Olga Gorodilina, p. 131: © Steph Adams, p. 132–133: © Courtesy of Hotel Arts Barcelona, p. 135: © Courtesy of Aria/Matt Moran, p. 138: Shutterstock.com/Paul Biryukov, p. 140–141: © Edible Material (Plant Café), p. 145: © Gabor Szantai, p. 146–147: © Bayleigh Vedelago, p. 150: © Edible Material (Plant Café), p. 152–153: © Courtesy of My Goodness, p. 155: © Rob Gilbert Photography, p. 156: © This is an extract from *I Quit Sugar: Simplicious* by Sarah Wilson, published by Pan Macmillan, RRP $39.99, p. 157: © Rob Palmer, p. 158: © Illustration by Megan Hess, p. 159: © Courtesy of Megan Hess, p. 172: © Chantell Bianchi, p. 173: (bottom) © Yie Sanderson Photography

Thanks to www.theblinkshop.co.za for wonderful props.
Very special thanks to Aliya Holland for cooking and food styling.

IMPRINT

© 2016 teNeues Media GmbH & Co. KG, Kempen

Texts by Tali Shine & Steph Adams

Editorial management &
photo editing by Regine Freyberg
Design & layout by Sophie Franke
Copy editing by Natalie Compton, Nadine Weinhold
Production by Nele Jansen
Imaging & proofing by David Burghardt/db-photo.de

Published by teNeues Publishing Group
teNeues Media GmbH + Co. KG
Am Selder 37, 47906 Kempen, Germany
Phone: +49 (0)2152 916 0
Fax: +49 (0)2152 916 111
e-mail: books@teneues.com

Press department: Andrea Rehn
Phone: +49 (0)2152 916 202
e-mail: arehn@teneues.com

teNeues Publishing Company
7 West 18th Street, New York, NY 10011, USA
Phone: +1 212 627 9090
Fax: +1 212 627 9511

teNeues Publishing UK Ltd.
12 Ferndene Road, London SE24 0AQ, UK
Phone: +44 (0)20 3542 8997

teNeues France S.A.R.L.
39, rue des Billets, 18250 Henrichemont, France
Phone: +33 (0)2 48 26 93 48
Fax: +33 (0)1 70 72 34 82

www.teneues.com

ISBN: 978-3-8327-3341-4
Library of Congress Control Number: 2015958061
Printed in Spain by Estellaprint

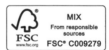